THE ULTIMATE GUIDE TO OVARIAN CANCER

The
Ultimate Guide
to
OVARIAN
CANCER

Everything You Need to Know
About Diagnosis, Treatment,
and Research

Benedict B. Benigno, M.D.

Sherryben Publishing House, LLC
ATLANTA, GEORGIA

Published by Sherryben Publishing House, LLC
Atlanta, Georgia

ISBN 13: 978-0-9887111-0-5

Library of Congress Control Number: 2012924261

First Sherryben Publishing House, LLC printing: January 2013

For my darling wife
Sheila

And my children
Justin
Alexander
Serena

And to
Northside Hospital

TABLE OF CONTENTS

AUTHOR TO READER

OVARIAN CANCER IS an avaricious tumor and its domain is nothing less than the entire abdominal cavity. It can extend from the deepest part of the pelvis up to the diaphragm and to the right and left of the colon and everything in between. It can appear after only a few weeks of the mildest symptoms and by then it has already declared *open season* on the body of a woman. It is fiendishly difficult to treat and unrelenting in its destructive ambition. It is a modern day scourge casting a narrow and selective net, forever changing the lives of its victims.

Ovarian cancer takes away from a woman health and dignity and presents her with a playing field that is far from level. While it is most common in women between the ages of 50 and 70, I have operated on patients as young as 16! As we shall see, this disease is not as silent as most people think it is. The symptoms are vague, do not always occur in the pelvis, and frequently masquerade as a gastrointestinal disorder. A careful history will reveal that more than 80 percent of these patients have symptoms.

Despite what you may have heard, there is no way to screen for ovarian cancer. A patient with advanced stage disease may present after weeks and sometimes only days of symptoms. However, a simple diagnostic test for this illness, one that can be done on a single drop of blood, that is inexpensive and 100 percent accurate, is one of oncology's Holy Grails. This book will explore the fact that the grail is not only holy, but near at hand.

Ovarian cancer will afflict more than 25,000 American women this year. It is one of the most difficult diseases to diagnose and the most lethal of all gynecologic malignancies. It is far more common in women who delay their first pregnancy until after the age of 35 or who do not ever become pregnant. It is seen more often in women who have a deleterious (harmful) mutation on the BRCA 1 or BRCA 2 gene, and yet only 10 percent of ovarian cancers are genetically linked. BRCA is an acronym for **BR**east **CA**ncer. It is a tumor suppressor gene, and so its damage will expedite the development of a cancer. The factors associated with this process are not well understood.

Patients almost always present with widespread metastases throughout the abdominal cavity, and the difficulties associated with the removal of all visible tumor challenge the most gifted and experienced of surgeons. The surgical procedure is invariably followed by heavy doses of chemotherapy and, as if that were not enough, the recurrence rate is between 70 percent and 80 percent! There is no other way to describe it— ovarian cancer takes a woman so far down that ground zero appears to be the heavens!

The process whereby a cell becomes malignant, eventually transposing the organ of origin into a clinical cancer, may ultimately prove to be far simpler than we have imagined. However, the mechanism whereby the cancer might be placed permanently into the past tense remains oncology's seemingly impossible dream. Some of my patients have expressed the notion that the cure for cancer has already been discovered, but is being suppressed by the pharmaceutical industry because cancer treatment is a multi-billion dollar industry. I reject this concept as wishful thinking. However, I am intrigued by the thought that, because the volume of cancer research is so staggering and is being performed by researchers working in such narrow intellectual spaces, perhaps work that could truly make a difference has not only been done already, but has also been published and remains unrecognized by those who could understand its significance and take it to a clinically relevant level.

A good example of this can be found in the antics of two researchers many years ago. Publish or perish is academia's great admonition. In an attempt to publish something, they took fifty chickens and removed the bursa of Fabricius, which is the outcropping present in the chicken's neck, to see what the result would be. Nothing happened to the chickens, so nothing was published. They decided to do another experiment in which the red blood cells of sheep were injected into a hundred chickens. They found that fifty of these chickens died and the other fifty went on as though nothing had happened to them. When they did their homework they discovered that they had made a laboratory error in that the original fifty chickens were included in the study.

In a research project such as this, all the animals should be equal; all of the chickens should have had the bursa of Fabricius removed or none of them. However, after closer analysis, they discovered that the only chickens that survived the injection of sheep red blood cells were the ones that had had the bursa of Fabricius removed in the original experiment. The researchers tried to publish this work in such prestigious journals as *Lancet* and the *New England Journal of Medicine*, but their efforts were rewarded with rejection letters.

The work was eventually published in the *Wisconsin Journal of Poultry Medicine*, a journal that I must confess I do not read on a regular basis. A researcher at the National Institutes of Health stumbled upon the article and immediately recognized its extraordinary value. The bursa of Fabricius in the chicken is the exact equivalent of the thymus gland in the human. The thymus gland is located in the upper part of chest in front of the heart and behind the sternum (breast bone). It is a very important part of the immune mechanism. The thymus gland must be suppressed when an organ is transplanted from a donor who is not an identical twin. These two men, whose only apparent reason for such research was to climb an obscure academic ladder, did nothing less than usher into modern medicine the era of transplant surgery. And their discovery almost went unrecognized!

Maybe the eventual cure for cancer will, in retrospect, appear ever so simple. I once heard Leonard Bernstein lecture. He sat down at the piano and played four notes—G-G-G-E flat, the famous opening of Beethoven's fifth symphony. He went on to say that the entire first movement of that symphony was but a combination and permutation of those four simple notes. And then, with a wry smile he said, "Anybody could have thought of that, of course, if you are Beethoven!" I hope that we will not have to wait for the scientific equivalent of a Beethoven to appear on the research stage in order to change the dreary paradigm that now constitutes the manner in which patients are treated for cancer.

This book will explore the exciting background of the development of a new diagnostic test for ovarian cancer, which we believe to be 100 percent sensitive and 100 percent specific. The reader will gain an insight into the diagnosis and treatment, as well as the devastation, of cancer using ovarian cancer as a model. I will explore novel treatments and attempt to acquaint the reader with the scientific background at the heart of clinical and basic science research. I will address frequently asked questions and make every attempt to present the science in language that is easily understandable.

We should remember that surgery and radiation therapy in the management of patients with cancer are now more than a hundred years old, and that chemotherapy has been around for almost seventy years. New and exciting basic research is being published on a daily basis. I hope that these new discoveries will soon lead to an era when oncologists do not have to slash, burn, and poison their way through yet another century. Perhaps in the near future some young physician will stumble across one of my operative reports and be amazed at the amount of surgery performed for what he or she would be able to treat with a simple vaccination! Polio no longer causes the fear it once did, and hopefully the terror that accompanies cancer will soon dissipate as revolutionary new-age treatments transpose even this disease into the realm of historic perspective.

I founded the Ovarian Cancer Institute twelve years ago and I serve as its chief executive officer. Professor John McDonald is the chief scientific officer and he directs all of the basic research of the Institute in his laboratory in the School of Biology at the Georgia Institute of Technology. The work is dedicated to the discovery of a highly accurate diagnostic test for ovarian cancer as well as to the development of better and less harmful forms of treatment. I think that the reader might enjoy a behind the scenes insight into the creation of a major cancer research unit as well as a glimpse into the financial and political problems that we encounter. Nothing, even in cancer research, is as simple as it appears to be.

Interwoven throughout this book will be a narrative of one woman's remarkable journey through the entire spectrum of ovarian cancer. In an effort to make the book more personal, the histories of many other memorable patients are described in detail. These histories are accurate and represent patients that I have cared for in my practice at Northside Hospital in Atlanta. Their names have been changed, and I hope that, in deference to their privacy, no effort will be made to uncover their identities. For the sake of convenience, I have used first names repetitively throughout the text. I would like the reader to know that I never address my patients by their first names. I always use their last names preceded by the title Ms. Not only does this indicate respect, but in my experience it contributes to the removal of barriers between patient and physician, especially since I use my first name when I introduce myself to them.

1

THE CANCER

And lo! the starry folds reveal
The blazoned truth we hold so dear
To guard is better than to heal, —
The shield is nobler than the spear!

THIS BOOK BEGINS with a quotation from an obscure poem by the legendary Supreme Court Justice Oliver Wendell Holmes. I think that it captures the very essence of medicine which is the prevention of disease rather than the development of difficult and harmful modalities of treatment. As we shall see, many patients can survive an advanced cancer but at a terrible price. In my entire four years in medical school there was not a single lecture devoted to the prevention of illness. The heroes were those who performed the longest and most difficult surgical procedures.

The Pap smear, which becomes positive before a cancer develops, is cervical cancer's shield that guards against the spear of surgery, radiation, and chemotherapy. However, there is no such shield for ovarian cancer. A woman may refuse a

Pap smear and risk developing an advanced cancer of the cervix. However, with respect to cancer of the ovary, she does everything correctly—an annual pelvic exam and Pap test and even a pelvic ultrasound and CA 125 blood test—and this dreadful cancer, which comes as a thief in the night, could change her life forever.

One of my most memorable patients flew to Atlanta from New York to consult for one of the large communication companies. At the end of the day she was dressing for dinner and became acutely short of breath. She went to the hospital where an x-ray showed that the left side of her chest was filled with fluid that tested positive for ovarian cancer cells. She had a Stage IV cancer of the ovary with only two hours of symptoms, and yet she had had a pelvic examination and Pap smear performed by her gynecologist just three months before this happened! It is very important to know that a routine annual pelvic examination will pick up an ovarian cancer only once in 10,000 visits!

The ovary is derived in the embryo from the genital ridge, the same tissue that produces the peritoneal lining (the thin membrane that lines the interior of the abdomen), which explains why primary peritoneal cancers are identical to ovarian cancers both visibly and microscopically. Fallopian tube cancers are also identical to ovarian cancers and are treated the same way. In fact, there is some interesting current research suggesting that all ovarian cancers may actually originate in the Fallopian tube.

Unlike cancer of the cervix, which is related to the HPV virus, and cancer of the lung, which is related to cigarette smoking, little is known about the origin of cancer of the ovary. The monthly ovulatory cycle produces an explosion in an ovary as the egg is released, and this appears to be why having pregnancies early in life may confer protection against this disease. Women almost never ovulate during pregnancy or during the time that they breast feed. If the first pregnancy is delayed until age 35, the damage of repetitive ovulation has already been done and pregnancy no longer exerts a protective effect.

It is believed that the damage to the ovary at the time of ovulation contributes to the genesis of this cancer. Following the rupture of the monthly cyst in the ovary that releases the egg (ovulation), epithelial cells (the cells which line the outermost part of the ovary) proliferate to repair surface damage. This phenomenon could occur twelve times a year for almost forty years. The birth control pill, which prevents ovulation, confers on the patient an extraordinary protection against ovarian cancer if it is taken for more than five years. In some cultures women get pregnant at the time of their first ovulatory cycle, breast feed for several years (which in itself prevents ovulation), and then have many subsequent pregnancies. These women may ovulate only ten or twelve times in a lifetime as opposed to twelve times a year in Western countries. In such cultures, cancer of the ovary is almost unheard of.

Women who take estrogen hormone without the addition of progesterone hormone will have a greater risk of ovarian cancer, as will patients with a strong family history of breast and ovarian cancer. Contrary to what was once believed, fertility drugs do not increase this risk. Ovarian cancer can occur in women who are in their 20s, but this is unusual. The older the patient is, the greater the risk, but this is true for almost all cancers.

Donald Woodruff, a famous pathologist at Johns Hopkins University many years ago, proposed an interesting theory regarding the origin of ovarian cancer. Unlike the body of a man, a woman's body has a direct conduit between the outside world and the interior of the abdomen. It was Dr. Woodruff's opinion that the granules from talc powder, used for generations during diaper changes, work their way into the abdomen via the vagina, cervical canal, uterine cavity and Fallopian tubes. When we examine the microscopic slides of patients with cancer of the ovary we frequently see large, calcified granules called psammoma bodies, making this theory very intriguing. In the absence of any other viable explanation except for repetitive ovulation, perhaps something as common and apparently harmless as talcum powder may contribute to the development of cancer of the ovary!

The highest incidence of this cancer is in the Scandinavian countries and the lowest incidence is in Asia. It is particularly prominent in women of Ashkenazi descent and if these women have a deleterious mutation on the BRCA 1 gene they have a **70 percent** chance of getting cancer of the ovary! The two BRCA genes are of enormous importance in the development of breast and ovarian cancer and they serve as a model for the genetic background in other cancers.

No other organ gives rise to as many different kinds of tumor as the ovary and no other organ produces tumors as large. The largest ovarian tumor on record weighed over 200 pounds and the largest that I have ever removed weighed in at 47 pounds. Although the ovary is involved in many types of tumor growth, this book will confine itself only to epithelial cancers which are the most common and which are derived from the surface or epithelial cells of the ovary.

More than 25,000 women in the United States will get cancer of the ovary this year and the overall survival is not a whole lot better than it was twenty years ago. With improvement in the surgical procedure as well as the development of newer chemotherapy regimens, there is a longer interval between diagnosis and death but little change in the overall cure rate. Another most dreary statistic is a recurrence rate of approximately 70 percent. Many of these women with recurrent ovarian cancer will eventually die of this disease. The life of such a patient can sometimes be prolonged for many years but at a terrible price, involving repetitive chemotherapy regimens and frequently additional surgery. Unlike cancers in other organs, no anatomic barrier (a covering, such as the capsule of the liver or the outer membrane of the bowel) exists to the spread of ovarian cancer. When first diagnosed, it has metastasized widely in most patients.

In his Pulitzer Prize-winning history of cancer, *The Emperor of all Maladies,* Siddhartha Mukherjee tells the story of the Persian Queen Atossa, whose cancerous breast was amputated by a slave. He brings her back in several parts of the book showing how her prognosis would have improved as advances in medicine occurred, but goes on to say that with some cancers, such as bile duct cancers, the prognosis would be the same today as it was 2,500 years ago. Unfortunately, even in the last twenty years the improvement in survival for many cancers has not been as good as anticipated.

Cancer of the ovary has a distinct biology and presentation at the clinical, cellular, and molecular levels. A complex cystic mass in the pelvis is the most common clinical occurrence. It is not the great *silent killer* that most people think it is. There are symptoms in more than 80 percent of cases, but these symptoms are generalized and frequently mistaken for other conditions, most often in the gall bladder and gastrointestinal tract. Cramping abdominal pain and bloating, along with fatigue and loss of appetite, are common presenting symptoms. If the ovarian tumor is large enough, it can press on the bladder, causing frequency of urination. Pressure on the rectum can produce bowel symptoms including constipation **and** diarrhea.

A detailed and highly accurate family history is a very important entry into a patient's chart, and that is never more important than in the case of a patient who has cancer. It is amazing how often the family history goes back only as far as the parents. A strong family history of uterine and colon cancer, as well as other gastrointestinal cancers, may indicate the presence of a syndrome known as hereditary nonpolyposis colorectal cancer (HNPPC), known as Lynch Syndrome. This syndrome is associated with a higher risk for the development of ovarian cancer.

Alcohol consumption does not seem to be related to the genesis of ovarian cancer, but, strangely enough, a Swedish study found that women who drink two or more glasses of milk a day have an increased risk of developing this cancer. Women who live in tropical climates have a lower rate of ovarian cancer, probably related to an increased exposure to vitamin D.

Although metastases can occur through lymphatic drainage to regional lymph nodes or via the blood stream to the liver or lung, the most common route the disease takes goes directly into the abdomen due to the sloughing off of the tumor cells from the outer surface of the ovary.

The cancer cells can block lymphatic channels and blood vessels, thus producing ascites, which is the accumulation of fluid in the abdomen. This is the way ovarian cancer frequently presents because the abdomen becomes markedly distended. The fluid can be drawn off by inserting a catheter into the abdomen under CT or ultrasound guidance. More than ten liters of fluid can accumulate and this is responsible for most of the fatigue and weakness that accompanies this disease. The fluid is not just water but contains precious proteins, electrolytes, and amino acids and this accumulation is a constant drain on the patient's nutritional status.

The imaging studies that will be mentioned throughout this book are the CT scan and the PET scan. CT refers to computerized axial tomography (CAT) and shows the body's structures, as well as the deformities produced by cancer, with remarkable clarity. A PET scan (Positron Emission Tomography) is identical to the CT scan except that a radioactive sugar molecule is injected intravenously prior to the scan. Since cancer cells consume increased amounts of sugar, such technology is helpful in determining whether a nodule is secondary to cancer or something else, such as an area of inflammation.

The cancerous areas will "light up" and the benign nodules will not. It is important that we all realize that this technology is not infallible. I have removed large lymph nodes that were positive on PET scan and found, to my surprise, that they were benign. On the other side of the spectrum, I recently operated on a patient whose PET scan was negative only to find a large, cancerous mass in the upper abdomen. Technology is a welcome and extraordinary adjunct to the work of an oncologist, but it is not a substitute for experience and clinical judgment.

Much work and a large amount of money have gone into the development of a diagnostic test for ovarian cancer. Such a test would save the lives of so many women and prevent an unspeakable amount of suffering and degradation. Only 20 percent of patients are diagnosed in Stage I. However, as previously noted, in more than 70 percent of patients the cancer has spread throughout the abdomen at the time of diagnosis. If the tumor can be discovered when it is in Stage I and is treated properly, the cure rate would be in excess of 90 percent! In more advanced stages the cure rate drops precipitously. The staging system for ovarian cancer is outlined below:

I.   Limited to one or both ovaries

    A.   One ovary, no ascites (abdominal fluid), capsule intact, no tumor on external surface

    B.   Both ovaries, no ascites, capsule intact, no tumor on external surface

    C.   One or both ovaries with ascites, ruptured capsule, tumor on surface or malignant cells in the peritoneal washings

II. Spread limited to the pelvis

    A.   Involvement of the uterus and or Fallopian tubes

    B.   Involvement of other pelvic tissues

III. Peritoneal implants above the pelvis and/or positive retroperitoneal or inguinal lymph nodes

    A.   Microscopic seeding of the abdominal peritoneum

    B.   Abdominal implants two centimeters or less

    C.   Abdominal implants greater than two centimeters

IV. Distant metastases

Cytoreductive surgery is a broad term that runs the gamut from removing the uterus, tubes, ovaries, and part of the omentum (the fat pad that hangs down from the stomach), to ultra radical procedures including the removal of the spleen and part of the colon, multiple small bowel resections, stripping of the diaphragm, and, in some cases, the removal of part of the diaphragm, partial liver resections, and the removal of the distal pancreas and lymph nodes. Ovarian cancer is one of the few tumors where such advanced surgery is performed because the cure rate is so much higher when all the cancer is removed. This allows subsequent chemotherapy to be more efficacious. The majority of patients will respond initially to a regimen of chemotherapy which includes Carboplatinum and Taxol.

It is not possible for even the most experienced of oncologists to predict the outcome in these patients. We have all seen women with early stage disease die within months of surgery and chemotherapy, whereas patients with the most advanced disease respond beautifully and get on with their lives as though nothing had ever happened. I will never forget the first patient that I treated with platinum chemotherapy well over thirty years ago. She was given the drug after a surgical procedure accomplished nothing because of the extent of disease in the upper abdomen. Following six courses of the platinum drug I re-operated on her, and, to my astonishment, the tumor had disappeared. What had been previously inoperable turned into one of the easiest operations that I have ever performed.

She was from the mountains of Tennessee, and, although I tried very hard to acquaint her with the seriousness of the situation, she put her trust in the treatment recommended and chose never to worry about it. Perhaps refusing to acquire knowledge about a lethal disease is one of the instruments of healing that is denied to those patients who spend ten hours a day at the computer learning everything that they can about ovarian cancer. Maybe Thomas Gray was right when he wrote " . . . where ignorance is bliss, / 'Tis folly to be wise."

The arrival of the chemotherapy drug Taxol on the scene was a major advance in the treatment of patients with ovarian cancer and soon became first-line therapy along with Carboplatinum. Taxol is now manufactured in the laboratory of a large pharmaceutical company, but in the beginning it was laboriously derived from the Pacific Northwest yew tree (*Taxus brevifolia*), the habitat of the Rocky Mountain spotted owl, and was very hard to come by. There were environmental groups protesting the cutting down of the yew trees and the endangerment of the owls.

During this difficult time when Taxol was rationed I came upon a truly unbelievable event on the oncology ward at Northside Hospital. I was writing on a chart when I saw one of my patients pacing up and down the corridor chanting, "No yews for Jews—no yews for Jews." I sat down with her and I told her that this was not personal—I had a great deal

of difficulty procuring this drug for Roman Catholics, South-
ern Baptists, and Muslims. I had the strange feeling that this
explanation was less than adequate and although the chanting
stopped, our relationship did not get back on track until there
was a shipment of Taxol with her name on it.

2

THE PATIENT

What it is like to be a woman, the irreconcilable difference of it—that sense of living one's deepest life underwater, that dark involvement with blood and birth and death.

—Joan Didion, *The White Album*

*I don't want to die. I want **not to be.***

—Marina Tsvetayeva
Twentieth-Century Russian Poet

DEATH IS AN abstract concept until its imminence slams into you. As many times as I have had conversations with my patients concerning end of life issues, I cannot imagine what it would be like to be on the receiving end of such a discussion. I love the metaphor of life as a banquet. If this is true then death is a rude interruption of a very important meal. I remember Saint Augustine's famous prayer, "Grant me chastity and continence, but not yet." A seriously ill person will bargain, in the beginning, for a few more years and then for weeks or even days. In D.M. Thomas' excellent book, *Eating*

Pavlova, the death of Sigmund Freud is described in graphic detail. He was suffering from terminal cancer of the jaw, which was producing intolerable pain, and emitting a stench that no one could abide, and yet, each morning he would say to his daughter Anna, "Not today—I will die tomorrow."

My patient Dana was bright, well educated, and a high-level executive with a large Atlanta corporation. She was in her 30s, recently married, and very much in control of her life. Like all young women, she thought that disease and death were problems that happened to others. She developed pain in the right lower part of her abdomen and underwent an appendectomy, at which time an advanced cancer of the ovary was found. This, unfortunately, is not unusual since ovarian cancer is frequently mistaken for other conditions.

The ovary is the only organ in the body that has its functioning cells facing the interior of the abdomen, and so, long before a tumor forms, malignant cells become detached and implant on the surfaces of the bowel, liver, and diaphragm, etc. The adhesiveness that allows the cancer cells to implant on these surfaces is complicated and not well understood at this time. It is the coalescence of these nodules, particularly around the bowel, that causes the patient's initial symptoms—bloating and cramping abdominal pain, especially after eating. These symptoms are, in effect, the symptoms of an early partial small bowel obstruction! It is not unusual for the only complaint to be, "My jeans are too tight and I am not gaining weight." To make matters worse, a decrease of these symptoms may occur and there may be some improvement until they return with a vengeance and become not only permanent but more intense.

A blood clot in the leg of a young woman is secondary to a cancer of the ovary until proven otherwise. Since some cancers wreak havoc with the body's complex clotting mechanisms, when a blood clot occurs, a pelvic ultrasound, CA 125 blood test, and a pelvic examination should be performed immediately. I have seen many cancers of the ovary present when the only finding was a blood clot in the leg.

Dana came into my office with a mixture of panic and confusion. There was a monotone quality to her voice and a faraway look in her eyes that said that she wanted to be anywhere else but in my office. She was missing her appendix, but a large amount of cancer remained in her abdomen. She wanted it out and wanted to get on with her life and expressed these wishes in very emphatic terms. A lengthy and dreary conversation ensued in which the surgical procedure, as well as all possible complications, were explained in graphic detail. She was offered a second opinion but she declined. The surgical procedure was scheduled.

In a well-run office a number of things happen after the surgery is scheduled, including lab work, x-rays, and, most importantly, a one-hour session with one of the nurses where everything that will happen from the moment she enters the hospital until the moment she is discharged, is explained in minute detail. All questions are answered. Since she had my cell phone number she could call me directly after the meeting with the nurse if any additional questions arose. In these situations knowledge is not only power—it is an instrument that lessens anxiety and induces a less terrifying optic. Medicine is first and foremost a communicative art. If I had known that as a young man I would have majored in English literature rather than biology.

Who has not stood in wonder at the almost painful beauty of frescoes painted on Italian ceilings? The ceilings on the way to the operating room, by contrast, are dreary in the extreme and constitute the patient's only view. I remember Dana staring in terror at the ceiling as the effects of the anesthetic transported her to another realm. At such a moment a well-intended remark, even if it is somewhat banal, can be of enormous comfort. At the last moment of apparent consciousness she was told that the A team was here and that we would take very good care of her. The door to the operating room closed and all remained silent as a nurse recited the *time out*—a review of the patient's name, diagnosis, and proposed operation for which a consent form had been signed—a further guard against needless error.

The operating room is as close to a controlled environment as a physician ever encounters. Everyone stops talking, the overhead lights are adjusted, an Angela Hewitt Bach recording is turned on, and the scrub nurse passes off a scalpel. This is the moment when it is very important that the surgeon disassociate himself or herself from the personhood of the patient and concentrate exclusively on the technical aspects of the procedure so that the operation may proceed in an environment uncontaminated by fear, or any other emotion. All of the cancer was removed and her recovery was swift and free from complication. She then received six courses of chemotherapy, which she tolerated remarkably well although she lost her hair.

She was able to work throughout the treatments, and, as she settled into the regimen, she actually became a source of strength and inspiration for the other patients around her. All treatment stopped within four months of our initial meeting and she went into what is known as a follow-up mode with office visits and lab work every three months and the occasional CT scan. Eventually, she was seen only every six months. Many years went by and since all modalities of testing remained negative we both thought that she was home free.

3

THE TEST—
EARLY
RUMBLINGS

*The art of medicine consists of amusing the patient
while nature cures the disease.*

—Voltaire

WOULDN'T IT BE wonderful to have a diagnostic test for ovarian cancer that would indicate the presence of the disease while it was still in Stage I or, better yet, before the surface ovarian cells actually become malignant? That is exactly what the Pap smear does—it becomes positive before the cervical cancer becomes invasive so that the treatment can be done in the office with a wire loop cautery (LEEP procedure). This removes the entire abnormality under microscopic guidance, allowing the uterus to remain, and makes subsequent pregnancies possible. With very rare exception, ovarian cancer takes away all possibility of pregnancy, and this is a particular tragedy since many of these women have never had a child.

There are some cancers for which a diagnostic test not only indicates the presence of the tumor, but acts as a barometer for the success of subsequent treatment. Gestational trophoblastic disease is a group of pregnancy-related diseases, which are occasionally highly lethal. This disease is treated until the HCG (human chorionic gonadotropin) blood test is negative. The HCG is the pregnancy test. Germ cell (primitive cells destined to become ova or eggs) tumors of the ovary can secrete HCG or AFP (alpha-fetoprotein), which not only help with the diagnosis of the condition but also allow a physician to evaluate the success of the treatment. Germ cell tumors of the ovary are quite rare, comprising less than 5 percent of all ovarian tumors. Ninety-five percent of ovarian cancers are epithelial in origin, and for these tumors there is no accurate diagnostic test.

The CA 125 blood test is by far the most common test used for ovarian cancer and many oncologists wish that it would just go away. It is a high molecular weight protein that measures an antibody. The test is neither sensitive nor specific. Sensitivity measures the proportion of positives (those people who actually have the disease), and specificity measures the proportion of negatives (the number of people who do not have the condition). A diagnostic test for ovarian cancer must be virtually 100 percent sensitive and specific; otherwise too many women with ovarian cancer will be missed and too many women who do not have ovarian cancer will be reported as positive.

The CA 125 test is elevated in 70 percent of patients with cirrhosis of the liver and 60 percent of patients with pancreatic cancer. Basically, it is a test for inflammation and may be positive in conditions as disparate as gall bladder disease and a urinary tract infection. As if that were not bad enough, 20 percent of patients with ovarian cancer have a negative CA 125. As you might imagine, both sensitivity and specificity are way off the mark and this test is absolutely useless as a diagnostic marker. The CA 125 has been around for more than thirty years and is frequently elevated in young women with endometriosis and fibroid tumors of the uterus, inducing terror in the patient and causing a never-ending series of tests and even unnecessary surgery.

The highest CA 125 levels that I have seen (well over 10,000) were found in patients with cirrhosis of the liver. Wouldn't it be nice to have a simple, highly accurate, and inexpensive test that would pick up an ovarian cancer at the earliest stage or even before the surface epithelial cells turn malignant—a test that along with the Pap smear would become part of the routine annual visit to the gynecologist? OVA 1 is a new blood test to detect ovarian cancer. It consists of a number of compounds in addition to the CA 125 protein. Another highly touted screening test, OvaSure, also includes the CA125 protein in its list of compounds. Both of these tests have an unacceptably low specificity rate and neither has passed into universal acceptance.

About twelve years ago I decided to limit my practice mainly to patients with cancer of the ovary. This allowed me to get involved in research trials and develop a referral center for women afflicted with this disease. It was about this time that I started the Ovarian Cancer Institute, which is dedicated to the development of a diagnostic test for ovarian cancer as well as to the discovery of more efficacious and less toxic forms of treatment.

Years before it was actually founded, it swam in my imagination. After awhile I realized that no one gives money to a dream; I had to raise the money myself. I received a lot of criticism for this decision from both colleagues and family, all of whom advised me that such work was already in progress at many major research centers that had access to considerable funding. I remained convinced that there was room for a research entity that was dedicated solely to ovarian cancer and was capable of *out-of-the-box* thinking.

The Institute began with a simple telephone call to John McDonald, who at that time was chair of genetics at the University of Georgia (UGA). I told him that I operate on many patients with cancer of the ovary and that their tissue and serum are wasted with respect to basic science research. I explained the dire need for a diagnostic test and I invited him to become the chief research scientist of the Ovarian Cancer Institute. We met at a restaurant in Atlanta and over a long dinner discovered that we had many things in common, including the survival of a Jesuit education.

He accepted the offer but told me that no work could begin until we acquired a microarray analyzer. This is an instrument that is capable of measuring the expression levels (i.e., the levels at which genes are "turned on" in cells) in all genes in the human genome. By considering differences in these expression patterns between cancer and normal precursor tissue (tissue from which the cancer may eventually arise), we would be able to identify those genes contributing to the cancer. The instrument, however, came with the hefty price tag of $250,000! When I asked him if that could be put into his department's budget for the coming year he simply smiled and withheld comment.

Not so long ago if a researcher wanted to measure the expression level of genes in a cancer, he or she would have to proceed one gene at a time, and since there are around 25,000 genes in a human cell a great deal of luck would have to ensue to make a significant discovery. With the microarray analyzer, all the genes are processed in multiple replicates on a microchip the size of a thumbnail and are analyzed in a computerized scanner attached to the unit. This would give us the enormous opportunity to build a database of genes differentially expressed between normal cells and ovarian cancer cells drawn from a large sample size, an absolute necessity if we were ever to discover a diagnostic marker. There remained, however, the annoying matter of the quarter of a million dollars.

Surgeons are not used to begging, but I had to make an exception when I walked into a local Atlanta bank. As I waited to see the manager, I thought of the famous story of Picasso, who had hosted a dinner party for some of his friends at a very expensive restaurant in the south of France in the 1920s. They were served exquisite food and vintage wines, and when the check, which bordered on extortion, was presented, Picasso simply sketched a picture of the restaurant's owner on the back of it, signed it and told him to keep the change! Every time that I have tried to do this the waiter asked me for plastic!

Was there some way that I could pull off a similar stunt at my bank? This fantasy quickly dissipated as I was introduced to the manager and told that I would have to personally guarantee the loan. I left the bank with the check in hand and a queasy feeling of impending financial doom. As I proceeded to drop the check off at the McDonald Laboratory, I came to the proverbial fork in the road. To the left was the laboratory and to the right was the Ferrari dealership. Time would tell that I made the right decision, but the temptation of the moment was overpowering!

Anyone who has ever tried to integrate a private research unit into the framework of a major university knows how difficult this can be. Both sets of attorneys schedule endless meetings and the university assigns numerous committees to oversee the process. The Ovarian Cancer Institute was extremely fortunate when it aligned itself with UGA. Karen Holbrook was the University's senior vice president and provost and was so excited about this relationship that she cut through all the red tape and saw to it that we began our work at UGA in record time.

There are advantages of a private cancer research institute over one that is based at a medical school department. A few weeks after John told me that we needed a microarray analyzer, it sat on its perch in his lab with several of the company's representatives teaching the laboratory personnel how to use it. Researchers at a university would have to submit such a request to the chairperson of the department who would put it into next year's budget where it all too frequently would be turned down. Now that we had the unit in place it was easy to begin the work.

Ribonucleic acid, or RNA, is the molecule used to measure gene expression. It is very fragile, so the tissue submitted for study must be handled properly from the very beginning. Before even clamping the blood supply to the tumor, I remove a piece of it and drop it into a canister of liquid nitrogen, which flash freezes the tissue, rendering the cellular molecules stable. It could be equally well studied on the day it was collected or a hundred years later.

As we will soon see, the Ovarian Cancer Institute transferred its laboratories from the University of Georgia to the Georgia Institute of Technology (Tech) when John McDonald was appointed to the chair of the School of Biology. This appointment came as a surprise to the both of us, since John had not applied for this position. This was an extraordinary blast of good luck that not even I could have imagined. The transfer of the Institute's laboratories to Georgia Tech allowed the scope of our work to mingle with many other intellectual and scientific pursuits at Tech, including bioinformatics, bio-engineering, and biochemistry.

Gary Schuster was the vice president and provost at Georgia Tech at the time and it was he who was responsible for John's appointment. He saw to it that the transfer of the Ovarian Cancer Institute from UGA to Tech was seamless, and he was also responsible for the considerable funding that accompanied our move. It is so good to have brilliant friends in high places! A brand new laboratory and considerable un-anticipated funding! This brought luck to the level of an art form. All that was expected of us at Tech was to discover an accurate screening test and to find better ways of treating ovarian cancer. It would soon be brought home to me that there is no such thing as a free lunch.

A new building was recently opened and it is located next to our laboratory. It is the nanotechnology building and its construction was, in part, supported by a gift from Bernie Marcus through the Marcus Foundation. With the advent of nanotechnology, matter can be manipulated on an atomic and molecular level with structures down to the size of a nanome-ter. To give you some idea of the scope of this work, a nano-meter is **one billionth** of a meter. Nanotechnology embraces fields of science as diverse as organic chemistry, molecular biology, and semiconductor physics. It is the integration of nanotechnology into the field of molecular biology that is so exciting in our work at the Ovarian Cancer Institute.

4

THE PHILOCTETES FACTOR

Philoctetes was a Trojan War hero who, prior to his involvement in the conflict, was bitten by a snake. This produced such a horrible, festering, and stinking wound that no one could abide his presence and he was banished to the uninhabited island of Lemnos.

THE STORY OF Philoctetes, subject of a little known play by Sophocles, is strangely relevant to the woman who has just been told that she has ovarian cancer. She feels like an outcast, that her life is coming to an end. She is enveloped by a strange sense of unworthiness, including, frequently, the loss of the perception of herself as a sexual being. Having a cancer in a sexual organ sometimes induces a sense of inadequacy with respect to sexuality that a cancer arising elsewhere does not.

These feelings frequently begin prior to the first office visit as instinct forms a prelude to reality.

I try to see to it that these patients are brought into my office immediately on arrival as a short interval in the waiting room reduces fear and builds confidence. I introduce myself without using the title of doctor and sit next to them and not behind a desk. These apparent small points remove barriers from an already fragile relationship and help the patient to believe that the healing process has begun.

What is the single most frightening moment in your life? I remember mine as though it were yesterday. I was asleep in my apartment in Saigon when the Viet Cong blew up the ammunition dump across the river, causing my bed to levitate briefly. Whatever it is that has frightened us in the past I am sure that, in most cases, it pales in comparison to hearing those dark words, "You have an advanced cancer of the ovary." Even if the diagnosis is anticipated, there is something about hearing it from the physician that confers not only finality but also the vision of impending doom. From that moment on the Sword of Damocles is hoisted above the patient's head and it is not removed until the treatment is over and a follow-up CT scan is negative. One of my patients who had a successful outcome told me that the sword was replaced by a pen knife. As Gilda Radner so eloquently put it, "It's always something."

Why are you here? I have found this simple question to be the best way to begin the relationship. Her answer gives me access to her understanding of the problem. It also informs me of her expectations as to how I might be able help her. Physicians, especially surgeons, are famous for interrupting their patients. The most difficult part of my day is listening to the patient's version of the development of the problem because I know it as well as she does. However, I have found that quietly listening to her is the best way to begin the relationship. Her narrative is very private and personal, and, despite its similarity to almost all other patients with cancer of the ovary, it is unique to her.

Following the physical examination, I sit down with the patient and her family, and, after making recommendations for treatment, I ask for questions. I have found that most husbands are very understanding and helpful but some are actually impediments to the healing process. They want to know if the cancer is contagious and some actually begin to tell me about *their* symptoms when I ask for questions. I am sometimes moved to write an article titled "Husbands I Have Known."

Both surgery and chemotherapy are important as one without the other dooms the patient to a recurrence. I try to imagine the mindset in the waiting room. Sadness and fragility go hand in hand at such moments, and, because most patients seek out the Internet before the office visit, confusion and terror walk into the office with them. Most of these women have had no symptoms until several weeks before the visit. They then come into my office and are told that they have ovarian cancer and that they will need extensive surgery and chemotherapy. Most shotguns have only two barrels! Computers give us data and accuracy but physicians give time and compassion. This is a huge passage in a woman's life and since the treatment is not an emergency, she should be offered the opportunity for another opinion. Such a recommendation on the part of the physician is a sign of confidence and goes a long way toward putting the patient at ease.

Another way to help jump start the relationship is to give her my personal cell phone number. Almost all communication is non-verbal and this apparently simple gesture sends the message that the physician is very interested in her return to health and a normal life. If a problem ensues she is going to reach me anyway, so why not make it easier for her by not making her call a voice prompt answering machine that instructs her to dial *one* for English, *two* for Spanish, *three* for Bulgarian, etc. I have found that far from causing needless intrusions into my time, patients armed with my cell phone number will actually try, sometimes to their detriment, *not* to call me. Access and communication are the very infrastructure of the art of medicine.

With respect to the opening question, I wonder if I am allowed to deviate from the text for a moment. Not all patients who come into my office have ovarian cancer. A well-dressed woman in her mid 20s came to see me for a most interesting problem. I asked her why she was here and her answer startled me. She told me that she was in a *platonic* relationship with a man who wanted to marry her. She went on to say that she knew that I was a very good surgeon and she wanted me to do an operation that would restore her *virginity!*

I have a very quick ear-brain synapse but I missed a beat or two prior to responding. I think that my answer was both urbane and sophisticated. I said something really brilliant such as, "Are you serious?" When she nodded in the affirmative I briefly wondered if this was why my mother sent me to medical school! And so, dear reader, what did I do? Did I tell her that I just wasn't that kind of surgeon, or did I take a piece of the chorionic plate from a newly delivered placenta, that part of the placenta that faces the baby, and using very fine plastic surgery sutures, stitch the membrane into the distal vagina thus giving her husband the illusion of a major deflowering? I think that I will downgrade this question to rhetorical status and leave it unanswered. Good gynecologists never talk!

5

THE OPERATION

Surgeons must be very careful
When they take the knife!
Underneath their fine incisions
Stirs the Culprit—life!

—Emily Dickinson

CONTRARY TO WHAT most people think, surgery is usually very easy to perform. The problem is to obtain the training and experience that allows it to be easy. I was very fortunate to have as my mentors two of the finest pelvic cancer surgeons that this country ever produced—John D. Thompson of the Emory University School of Medicine in Atlanta and Felix N. Rutledge of M.D. Anderson Hospital in Houston. They were vastly different men: Thompson was mercurial and excitable, especially in the operating room, and Rutledge was quiet, soft spoken, and given to barely perceptible sarcastic innuendo. Both men emerged from the Department of Obstetrics and Gynecology at the Johns Hopkins University School of

Medicine and trained a generation of pelvic cancer surgeons. Although they have not operated in more than twenty-five years, stories about them still resound at our annual medical meetings.

I worked with them after I finished my residency training and I remember how astonished I was at their skill and clinical acuity. Assisting them in the operating room and later being assisted by them were memorable moments in the life of a young surgeon. Tissue planes opened with apparent ease and the cancers actually appeared to be afraid of these two giants! Both men imbued in me a deep and abiding respect for the fear and pain that accompanies a patient's battle with cancer.

But as good as my training was under these two men, I have learned that the evolution of a surgeon's education does not end with the completion of a residency or fellowship training program—it is a lifetime pursuit, and a variety of experiences serve to enrich that pursuit. Prior to settling down in my first appointment as director of gynecologic oncology at Emory, I did something that provided one of those enriching experiences. I accepted the position of visiting professor at the University School of Medicine in Saigon, South Vietnam. I was there from 1970 to 1973, and, although it was during the war, it was a lot safer than the area in New York City where I grew up! My job was to set up a residency program in obstetrics and gynecology, which would train young Vietnamese surgeons in this specialty the way American physicians are trained.

I worked at the famous Tu Du Maternity Hospital. This was an old French colonial structure, which had well-equipped operating and delivery rooms. The place where women in labor were kept prior to delivery was a vast open room, and, since there were between 100 and 125 deliveries a day, the room was always filled. This hospital served as a referral center for interesting and difficult surgical procedures for a large part of South Vietnam, and during those three years I did an enormous amount of surgery. This served to build confidence as well as technical expertise. What began as a one-year visit lasted for three and proved to be among the most interesting junctures in my career.

The operating room is the proper domain of the gynecologic oncologist, and unfortunately, it is the *stopping-off place*, at least once, for all patients with cancer of the ovary. Prior to making the incision, I trace a line on the abdomen with a sterile marking pen that has a very fine point so that the incision is as straight and centered as possible. The skin is closed with a fine plastic surgery suture, which usually produces a hairline scar. One of my teachers once told me that the abdominal wound was my signature and that I should have very good handwriting.

As I have settled into my career as a surgeon, I have discovered that few things fill a room with a more eerie silence then a scalpel opening the anterior abdominal wall. As many times as I have done this, I continue to marvel at the sheer extent of the disease process unfolding before me. How can so much cancer exist in a body and produce so few symptoms until only weeks prior to surgery? Why are Stage III and IV cancers the rule whereas an encounter with a Stage I tumor is almost always a serendipitous event? To remove all visible cancer may take many hours, and, since some of these patients are elderly, great care must be expended in their preparation for surgery. Even in the most well-worked-up patient there are times when the surgical procedure must be abandoned and rescheduled after several courses of chemotherapy. Surgery is relatively easy to learn but wisdom comes with many years of work and with great difficulty.

In surgery, often the first thing that one sees, in addition to a mass in the ovary, is the presence of tumor nodules on the surface of the bowel and a large deposit of tumor on the omentum, which is the fat pad that hangs down from the stomach. A cancer in the ovary may vary from a normal-size ovary to one that weighs in excess of 20 pounds. I have seen Stage IV cancers when the ovary is normal in size, to give you some insight into how difficult it can be to diagnose this problem. There can be sheets of tumor enveloping the bladder and rectum. The undersurface of the diaphragm is a favorite resting place for these cancerous masses, as is the capsule of the liver. Unfortunately, this is far from an exhaustive list as the interior of the entire abdominal cavity is at risk and no operation for an ovarian cancer is complete unless a thorough visual and manual examination of the abdomen has been performed.

Parts of the surgical procedure for advanced cancer of the ovary can be quite dangerous, as the dissection of the cancer prior to its removal can be perilously close to such structures as the spleen, pancreas, kidney, and liver. For the experienced surgeon, such tumors can be removed with considerable safety and often without the need for a blood transfusion. It is extremely important that a well-trained and experienced gynecologic oncologist perform this procedure. General gynecologists are not trained to do these operations.

The most common finding in patients with cancer of the ovary is a mass in the pelvis. An ovarian mass can be of considerable size and produce no symptoms whatsoever. I was recently summoned to the emergency room to evaluate a 40-year-old woman who had an ovarian tumor the size of a large honeydew melon. I found it interesting that she was totally unaware of the *alien* in her body. She had gone to the emergency room because of a headache and a very astute nurse asked her if she was pregnant.

One should always presume that a large mass in the ovary is a cancer and see to it that the appropriate work-up is performed, This should include a CT scan of the pelvis *and* abdomen. It is important that the surgeon knows that everything else is normal so that there will be no surprises during surgery. Many years ago I would have operated on a woman for a pelvic mass had I not obtained a preoperative CT scan. The mass I had palpated turned out to be a normal kidney that had rotated down into the pelvis! That would have produced a rather interesting pathology report and since , rarely, a pelvic kidney is the patient's only kidney, tragedy could have been added to error.

As surgery for cancer of the breast has gravitated from the ultra-radical of generations ago to procedures as minimally invasive as a lumpectomy, surgical procedures for cancer of the ovary are becoming more extensive with each passing year. It is not uncommon for the undersurfaces of the diaphragm to be stripped or even removed, parts of the liver and pancreas resected, and the spleen removed. A large ovarian cancer may require extensive dissection in the pelvis with multiple bowel resections before it can be removed in its entirety. The recovery from such extensive surgery can be prolonged and complicated, thus delaying, sometimes for many weeks, the administration of chemotherapy, which is of equal importance to the surgical procedure. There is an ongoing debate regarding the use of preoperative chemotherapy to shrink the tumors and lessen the extent of the surgery. Like most debates in medicine, there are fierce proponents on both sides of the issue.

The postoperative care of these patients can be complicated and it is very important that they be sent to a ward where there are skilled nurses well trained in the care of patients with gynecologic malignancies. Atlanta's Northside Hospital has a large gynecologic oncology unit that is dedicated to the complete management of these patients. The unit includes not only skilled nurses but also counselors and navigators. All surgeons encounter post-operative complications—the secret is to recognize the problem and correct it properly and immediately. One of the factors that contributes to the early recognition of a complication is the presence of a caring and well-trained nurse. The only way to avoid a complication is to not do the operation, to open the abdomen and decide that the procedure would be too difficult or dangerous, the so-called peek and shriek operation!

While surgery has certainly advanced a good deal over the past few decades, it is important that a knowledge of history informs us of the courage of both surgeons and patients several generations ago. Surgery for ovarian tumors, for example, has one of the most unique stories in the entire history of medicine.

In 1809 Jane Todd Crawford lived in a small hamlet some sixty miles from Danville, Kentucky. This was Daniel Boone country and Danville was not exactly a thriving metropolis. She was being cared for by a local physician for what was presumed to be a pregnancy, but after ten months had gone by it was decided to summon Ephraim McDowell, who was an Edinburgh, Scotland–trained surgeon practicing in Danville. Ms. Crawford had an abdomen the size of a term pregnancy with twins and when Dr. McDowell examined her he pronounced the uterus to be empty and correctly diagnosed an ovarian tumor. This was done without the benefit of a CT scanner or an ultrasound unit. To put this into perspective, 1809 was the year in which Beethoven composed his fifth symphony, Napoleon occupied Vienna, and Abraham Lincoln was born. No one had ever survived the removal of such a tumor.

Dr. McDowell told Ms. Crawford that if she came to Danville he would try to remove it. She accepted his offer and rode the 60 miles to Danville on horseback, fording several rivers in the dead of winter with her enormous abdomen bouncing up and down on the saddle horn. He operated on her in an upstairs bedroom in his home on Christmas day assisted by his nephew, who begged him to abandon the procedure up until the very moment that the incision was made. He removed the tumor in twenty-three minutes, losing very little blood. He closed the abdomen under extremely hazardous conditions, as there was no anesthetist to administer drugs to relax the abdomen or to alleviate pain.

We should remember that this operation was performed many years before Crawford Long discovered the use of ether to relieve the pain of surgery. It was necessary for four strong men to hold her down since several shots of bourbon had not completely knocked her out. It was reported that she sang hymns and recited psalms to calm herself during what must have been an unimaginably terrifying experience. Several days later she was up and about, making her bed and tolerating a diet. She not only lived another thirty-three years but she also outlived her famous surgeon by twelve years!

So many things are taken for granted today—a tray of sterile instruments and an anesthesiologist for starters. I published a paper on the 200th anniversary of this operation. It was subtitled "The Bicentennial of a Surgical Masterpiece." I visited Dr. McDowell's home in Danville and stood in wonder at his accomplishment. We need to remember that this was not a teaching hospital in Paris or London. It was an upstairs bedroom in a Kentucky backwater. The surgeon was inventive and daring but the patient was very, very brave. Just for the record, it was noted during surgery that there were severe contusions of the abdominal wall caused by the constant banging of her massive abdomen on the saddle horn. You may be interested to learn that the same horse took her back home.

6

THE COMPLICATIONS

The first public obligation is to avoid extremes of suffering.

—Sir Isaiah Berlin
The Crooked Timber of Humanity

ONE OF MY most memorable teachers told me that my chief obligation as a surgeon was to keep my patients out of the operating room unless absolutely necessary. I think that there were two reasons for that mandate: Operating rooms will always be dangerous places and even the simplest of procedures can be associated with the most devastating complications. Since complications occur in the hands of the best and most famous surgeons, it behooves you to keep this in mind and become proactive if you feel that something is going wrong. It is not at all unusual for the patient to be the first person to call attention to a post-operative complication.

All possible known complications should be explained in their entirety by the surgeon or the staff before the operation. This conversation can be somewhat frightening, but it does prepare you for what lies ahead. This educational process may serve to alert you to problems before they become major issues. There is nothing wrong with asking a few important questions prior to surgery. Who is responsible for my care at night? Who will see me over the weekend? How can I reach you if something goes wrong?

This is how I teach medical students and residents during morning rounds so they can discover whether patients are experiencing any problems. You can apply this information to your own situation so that you can learn what the various symptoms mean. Most important, you must always discuss them with your doctor.

The phrases will be short and devoid of adjectives and dangling participles. Please imagine a surgeon in a white coat with several medical students and residents in tow. We are about to visit a patient who has had extensive surgery for cancer of the ovary four days earlier. The first thing that we are going to do is to knock on the door because this is her temporary home, and then we are going to say, "Good Morning!"

Does she have a fever? An elevation of the temperature can accompany all of the complications listed in this chapter and it is sometimes the first sign of a major problem. A fever that occurs within the first twenty-four hours following surgery is almost always due to pulmonary (related to the lungs) problems. A fever after the first postoperative day and within the first week is frequently due to an infection in the operative site. Spiking fevers (alternating between high and low) can be a sign of a serious infection such as an abscess.

Is the pulse high? This is frequently due to anxiety but can be the first sign of a serious postoperative complication such as:

- Blood loss
- Pneumonia
- Pulmonary embolus (blood clot to the lung)
- Wound infection
- Wound dehiscence (separation along the suture line)
- Sepsis (problems associated with a blood infection)
- Heart arrhythmias
- Injury to the ureter (the tube bringing urine to the bladder)
- Thyroid problems

Is she breathing rapidly (tachypnea)? This apparently minor issue can be a harbinger of disaster. A pulmonary embolus can occur in the absence of symptoms, but rapid breathing is the first physical sign of this disorder. Pneumonia can also present this way.

Look at her eyes—Have the whites of the eyes turned yellow, indicating jaundice? Is the tissue inside the lower eyelid pale, indicating anemia? Are the pupils equal—inequality can be a sign of a stroke? Are the eyes popping out (exophthalmos), indicating a thyroid problem?

The neck is a frequently overlooked structure. Are the neck veins distended? This can be a sign of a massive pulmonary embolus even if the pulse and blood pressure are normal and she appears OK. Is the neck stiff due to meningitis? If there is redness in the neck near a central intravenous line? This may indicate an early infection.

Listen to the lungs. Are breath sounds absent on one side of the chest? The possible causes of this are:

- Pneumonia
- Atelectasis (collapse of the lung)
- Pleural effusion (fluid in the chest)
- Pulmonary embolus
- Pneumothorax (air in the chest causing the collapse of a lung)

Examine the abdomen. There should never be a bandage covering the wound after the first postoperative day, thus allowing everyone, including the patient, to see it. The problems that one may encounter in the inspection of the abdomen include:

- Redness and swelling of the incision may indicate an infection

- Is there generalized swelling? This may be due to an ileus (temporary paralysis of the bowel), or an obstruction of the bowel

- Is there a clear, blood-tinged drainage coming from the incision? This frequently accompanies a wound dehiscence (opening of the incision)

Is there a constant drainage of fluid from the vagina? This can be caused by several conditions:

- An operative injury to the bladder or ureter

- Ascites (fluid in the abdomen) can reform and leak out of the vagina

Is there CVA (costovertebral angle) tenderness? This refers to pain in the upper side of the back and may indicate a kidney infection or an obstruction of the outflow tract of the kidney.

Is there pain or burning on urination? This may be due to irritation of the bladder from the previous catheter but sometimes it may indicate a serious urinary tract infection

Does she have diarrhea? This should never be taken lightly. Diarrhea can be a symptom of a bowel obstruction. It can also be due to pseudomembranous enterocolitis secondary to an infection with the bacteria known as *Clostridium difficile.* This serious problem needs to be treated immediately or it can result in the loss of the colon or even death.

No visit to a postoperative patient is complete without a careful examination of the legs. Some of the things that we look for are:

- Swelling! Is there a DVT (deep venous thrombosis or blood clot)?
- Is she in congestive heart failure?
- Absent arterial pulses in the foot and ankle
- Is one leg colder than the other possibly indicating a problem with blood supply?
- Is there a problem with leg motion? Nerve injury? Stroke?

It is very important for everyone to realize that a life-threatening emergency may emerge in the immediate post-operative period that has nothing to do with the operation that has just been performed. For instance, a pain in the right upper part of the abdomen, especially if it is accompanied by fever, may be due to an acute inflammation of the gall bladder. A pain localized in the right lower part of the abdomen may be due to appendicitis!

An experienced clinician will be able to differentiate normal postoperative tenderness from an acute abdomen (a very serious condition frequently requiring immediate surgery). If there is any doubt, a CT scan will be done to rule out not only the conditions just mentioned, but also such things as a bowel perforation or necrosis (dead bowel due to loss of blood supply). As you might imagine, both of these conditions are unusual but they are surgical emergencies of the very first magnitude.

This is a list of the most common complications encountered following surgery for cancer of the ovary. This chapter was written to inform and not to frighten. Most people who have abdominal pain and bloating do not have cancer of the ovary. Likewise, most people who have a fever and a high pulse rate after surgery do not have the complications listed above. Serious postoperative complications are not very common and almost all of them, if treated immediately and properly, have an excellent outcome with no long-term problems.

With considerable trepidation, I will tell you about one of the strangest and most frightening postoperative complications that I have ever encountered. I was a senior medical student at the time, and eight days had elapsed since this patient's abdominal operation. The abdomen remained distended and there was no bowel function. I ordered an abdominal x-ray and what I saw was truly amazing. There was an open, ten inch pair of steel scissors in the abdomen with the points abutting the liver! I asked the patient not to cough for fear of the scissors closing and cutting something.

Needless to say, I let the professor handle that one. He removed the scissors and the patient went home several days later without further problem. She is probably still talking over the Thanksgiving turkey about the great surgeon who saved her life, twice! This gives all of us an insight into what can go horribly wrong without producing a lasting effect. Need I add that this was an extremely unusual occurrence?

Whenever the abdomen remains distended for a prolonged period of time, a foreign body should be considered and an x-ray obtained. The most common object left in the abdomen after surgery is a lap pad, which is a small white towel used to keep the bowel away from the field of dissection. It should be noted that whenever a foreign body has been left in the abdomen, the counting that was done prior to taking the patient out of the operating room is always reported as correct! This is very scary and is why I always count everything again myself. After all, the buck stops with me.

Careful attention to the possibility of a postoperative complication should not end when you leave the hospital. All of the problems that I have mentioned can begin after you are discharged. Since you are away from the comfort zone of your health care team, certain issues can be more frightening than they would have been during your hospitalization. One of the most common postoperative complications to begin at home is bleeding. It is not uncommon to have vaginal bleeding begin several weeks after a hysterectomy. This is almost always due to the absorption of the stitches that were used to close the upper part of the vagina and should be of no concern unless the bleeding is heavy. An occasional phone call to your doctor's nurse is frequently all that it takes to assuage these anxieties. The body is a marvelous reparative instrument, but healing takes time.

7

THE DRUGS

Normality is a tightrope walker above the abyss of abnormality.

—Witold Gombrowicz
Ferdydurke

IT'S ALL ABOUT division! Cells divide and produce new daughter cells along strict guidelines and according to an internal timetable. There are several important phases in cell division. The S phase is where DNA synthesis occurs and the M phase is where mitosis (division) occurs. Cancer cells must divide far more rapidly than normal cells and so the cancer daughter cells divide before they have reached functional maturity. Chemotherapy drugs work by inhibiting DNA synthesis and slowing down mitotic cell division. The drugs slow down the division of normal cell also, but cancer cells are far more sensitive to this process. If cancer cells were to acquire a slogan I am certain that it would be, *divide and conquer!*

In a review titled "The Hallmarks of Cancer," published in the scientific journal *Cell*, Douglas Hanahan and Robert Weinberg provide an extraordinary insight into the complex mechanisms whereby a cancer cell develops. They suggest that this process is analogous to Darwinian evolution in which a succession of genetic changes leads to the conversion of a normal cell into a cancer cell. They have outlined six essential alterations in cell physiology that collectively program malignant growth transformation:

1. **Self-Sufficiency in Growth Signals**—Normal cells require inherent growth signals before they can proliferate. No normal cell can divide in the absence of such stimulatory signals The hallmark of a cancer cell is its ability to generate its own growth signals, thereby initiating growth independent of the processes that bind the proliferation of the normal cell.

2. **Insensitivity to Antigrowth Signals**—There are multiple anti-proliferative signals that operate within normal tissue and are responsible for normal tissue stability. By a number of mechanisms, some of which are not well understood, a cancer cell is able to evade these anti-proliferative signals with remarkable ease.

3. **The Evasion of Apoptosis**—Apoptosis is programmed cell death and this process of self-immolation is inherent in all normal cells. An acquired resistance to apoptosis is a unique quality in all cancer cells and confers on such cells an unfortunate immortality.

4. **Limitless Replicative Potential**—These three acquired capabilities (growth signal autonomy, insensitivity to antigrowth signals, and resistance to apoptosis) lead to an

uncoupling of a cell's growth program from signals in its environment. This causes the development of vast cell populations that eventually constitute a visible tumor.

5. **Sustained angiogenesis**—The oxygen and nutrients supplied through blood vessels are necessary for cell function and survival. Angiogenesis is the process whereby new blood vessels are generated and this process is absolutely necessary if cancer cells are to proliferate and a tumor grow.

6. **Tissue Invasion and Metastasis**—The capacity for invasion and metastasis enables cancer cells to escape the primary tumor site and invade other organs. This process can occur through the bloodstream, through lymphatic drainage, or, as is so frequently seen in ovarian cancer, by direct extension into organs within the abdominal cavity. The capacity for metastatic spread of a cancer is an extremely complex mechanism and remains a mystery.

These six unique forces present to the oncologist a formidable and terrifying opponent. Next to such opposition, how feeble and ineffective are the current modalities of treatment for any cancer, especially one that has metastasized to the liver and lung! We have yet to be able to intercept malignant cell proliferation at the signaling pathway level, which represents the next wave of cancer treatment prior to the eventual replacement of the oncologist by the molecular biologist.

Chemotherapy is the glove on the hand of surgery as it is very unusual for a patient with ovarian cancer to be told that she does not need postoperative treatment. The tumor would need to be confined to one ovary and be removed without rupture and a full staging procedure prove to be negative for any spread. It is hard to imagine now because of the pervasiveness of the treatment, but the history of chemotherapy goes back only to the late 1940s.

The very first time that a solid tumor was cured with chemotherapy was accomplished with a drug called methotrexate, and, although this drug is useless in the treatment of ovarian cancer, it has a unique history and has entered the lives of women on several different occasions. I think that it would be good to explore the evolution of this drug as a prelude to the discussion of chemotherapy for ovarian cancer.

In the 1930s Lucy Mills was a missionary physician. While working in Bombay (now Mumbai), India, she noticed that a vitamin B-rich yeast extract called Marmite could cure megaloblastic anemia not only in rats but also in pregnant women. Megaloblastic anemia occurs when there is inhibition of DNA synthesis in the red blood cells. The active ingredient responsible for this cure turned out to be folic acid, a member of the vitamin B compounds, and this was eventually extracted from spinach. Sidney Farber, the famous pediatrician working at the Massachusetts General Hospital in the 1940s, used this drug in the treatment of children with leukemia. He found that not only did the leukemia not regress, but the drug actually accelerated the leukemic process. This led him to believe that a folic acid antagonist might be the answer.

Folic acid was first synthesized in 1943 at the Lederle Laboratories in New York. Four years later they developed the folic acid antagonist drug aminopterin, and in that same year, 1947, Sidney Farber used this drug to produce the first remissions of acute lymphoblastic leukemia in children. Aminopterin is methotrexate and several years later it entered the specialty of gynecology with startling results.

In the early 1950s Roy Hertz and Min Chiu Li were working at the Sloan Kettering Memorial Hospital in New York City where they encountered a 24-year-old woman with advanced metastatic choriocarcinoma. This disease is the most serious form of a group of diseases called gestational trophoblastic disease.

Choriocarcinoma usually occurs after a molar pregnancy, which is a pregnancy in which the placenta grows in the absence of a fetus. However, the most serious form of the disease occurs following a normal pregnancy and delivery. Metastatic choriocarcinoma used to have a 100 percent mortality rate. Hertz and Li treated this patient with methotrexate and were astonished to see her recover and leave the hospital after four months of treatment She went on to lead a normal life and this rare and fatal cancer never recurred! The cure rate for gestational trophoblastic disease with the use of methotrexate regimens currently approaches 100 percent.

An ectopic pregnancy is a pregnancy that occurs outside of the uterus, usually in the Fallopian tube, and, although it is a benign condition, it is responsible for many deaths each year. In 1982 Toshinobu Tanaka first reported on the use of methotrexate in the treatment of an ectopic pregnancy. Prior to this the only treatment was surgery, which usually resulted in the loss of the Fallopian tube. With the use of trans-vaginal ultrasonography and the quantitative beta HCG level (pregnancy test), the diagnosis of an early ectopic pregnancy can be made with high accuracy and this condition can now be treated without surgery. Although it cannot be used in the treatment of ovarian cancer, methotrexate has made an extraordinary difference in the lives of many women.

Some of the drugs currently given to patients with cancer of the ovary are listed below:

- Carboplatinum (Carboplatin)
- Paclitaxel (Taxol)
- Docetaxel (Taxotere)
- Pegylated Liposomal Doxorubicin (Doxil)
- Topotecan (Hycamtin)
- Gemcitabine (Gemzar)
- Etoposide (VP-16)
- Xeloda (Capecitabine)
- Bevacizumab (Avastin)
- PARP inhibitors
- Arimidex (Anastrozole)
- Tamoxifen (Nolvadex)

Carboplatinum and Taxol are the two drugs that are given in first-line treatment. Doxil, Topotecan, and Gemzar are drugs commonly used for recurrences, either alone or in combination with another drug. One must always remember that these drugs are poisons and the dose and the interval between treatments depend entirely on the body's ability to withstand this repetitive poisoning. When Carboplatinum and Taxol are given to newly diagnosed patients, the route of administration depends on whether or not all of the cancer was removed. If there is no residual disease after surgery then many oncologists prefer to administer the chemotherapy directly into the abdominal cavity which is called the intraperitoneal (IP) route. If any tumor remains after surgery the drugs are administered intravenously. In many centers throughout the world the intraperitoneal route is considered standard of care. However, in some large and highly respected institutions the chemotherapy drugs are always given intravenously. Ovarian cancer remains a disease in search of a consensus.

If the intraperitoneal route is chosen, then a port is placed in the abdomen at the time of surgery. This device is a small round plastic receptacle with a silicone rubber catheter attached to it. The port is placed just beneath the skin and the rubber catheter lies within the abdominal cavity. The infusion needle is placed through the skin directly into the port and it is removed as soon as the IP treatment is finished. The IP regimen also includes the use of Taxol with a platinum agent and frequently Taxol is given intravenously as well as directly into the abdomen. Six courses usually constitute a complete treatment cycle but no one ever knows the appropriate time to stop therapy. The correct answer is that treatment should be stopped when the last cancer cell has been destroyed but at the present time this is unknowable.

Unless the patient has extraordinary veins, a chest port should be inserted. This resembles the intraperitoneal port, but its catheter lies within a large vein near the heart. When the infusion needle is placed into the device, there is immediate access to the venous system, preventing a spillage of chemotherapy into surrounding tissues. This would cause a terrible inflammatory reaction with redness, pain, and swelling that could last for months. An interventional radiologist can insert the chest port in an outpatient setting, interdicting the need to go to the operating room.

The difficulty lies in the management of a patient whose cancer recurs following first-line chemotherapy because there is no unanimity of opinion as to the best way to proceed. If there is a recurrence a year or more after the initial chemotherapy has stopped, I prefer to give Carboplatinum again and substitute Doxil for Taxol. However, there are many different regimens as well as several clinical trials available in this setting and a discussion with your physician is the best way to find the treatment that is most appropriate for you.

Desperately needed at this time is a form of maintenance therapy designed to eliminate or greatly reduce the chance for a recurrence—something well tolerated with few if any side effects. Maintenance therapy refers to treatment given immediately after the standard chemotherapy regimen has been completed. We used to give monthly Taxol at a reduced dose for a year, but this has fallen out of favor. As you might imagine, when there are so many active drugs for a single cancer, there is no one regimen on which everyone agrees.

The greatest problem that I face when I am treating a patient with a recurrent cancer of the ovary is the timing of the decision to stop the treatment. Exactly when is enough really enough? We all know that when a patient develops a recurrence she has an overwhelming chance of developing yet another recurrence. Is six months of treatment sufficient? How about a year? Where is the science in all of this? It is a very good sign to see the CA 125 level drop to normal but that does not mean that the last cancer cell has been destroyed. To add to the confusion and agony, even the PET scan will not pick up small nodules of recurrent tumor.

Carboplatinum is unique among drugs given for ovarian cancer in that it is excreted by the kidney rather than the liver. It is capable of causing serious kidney toxicity if the dosage is not carefully calculated. It can also cause hearing loss due to damage of the eighth cranial nerve. Both Carboplatinum and Taxol will cause hair loss and temporary bone marrow toxicity, which lowers the white blood cell count, red blood cell count, and platelet count sometimes to dangerously low levels. Transfusions of red blood cells and platelets may become necessary, and if the white blood cell count drops low enough, a dangerous blood infection called septicemia may develop. This requires hospitalization and the administration of powerful antibiotics. Medications are now available to raise the red and white blood cell counts, but nothing can raise the platelet count except a platelet transfusion.

There are many drugs available to combat nausea and this problem is not nearly as bad as it used to be. Both Carboplatinum and Taxol can produce a peripheral neuropathy manifested by numbness and tingling and sometimes pain in the hands and feet. This can be very severe and it may sometimes be necessary to discontinue the treatment and substitute another regimen. Gabapentin (Neurontin) is used to combat the neuropathy and the administration of vitamin B6 may sometimes mollify these symptoms. The side effects in some patients can be so severe that I sometimes wonder if the treatment might be worse than the disease.

Bevacizumab or Avastin (its commercial name) is a vascular disruptive agent, one that interferes with blood vessel production. It is now used in the management of recurrent ovarian cancer, either alone or in combination with a chemotherapy drug. Avastin is not chemotherapy; rather, it is a monoclonal antibody that inhibits vascular endothelial growth factor (VEGF). The endothelium is the layer of cells that line blood vessels and a drug that can block the cancer's ability to make new blood vessels will not only cause the tumor to shrink, but will also reduce the accumulation of fluid in the abdomen and chest.

Since Avastin is not chemotherapy, it has none of the side effects of chemotherapy such as hair loss, bone marrow depression, peripheral neuropathy, etc. However, this drug has its own set of side effects that are sometimes so severe that the drug must be stopped. Nosebleeds, changes in blood pressure, and an increase in the excretion of protein in the urine are seen often. A pseudo-encephalopathy syndrome, which mimics a stroke, can occasionally occur. By far, the most serious complication seen with Avastin is a bowel perforation. Sometimes the tumor nodules on top of the bowel dissolve so rapidly that an opening occurs in either the small or large intestine.

Most patients taking Avastin have had a number of previous surgical procedures and so the bowel leakage may be contained within abdominal adhesions and not require emergency surgery. The bowel contents can spontaneously drain through the skin, forming a self-induced opening in the abdominal wall, which can be bagged, like a colostomy, until it closes. It is also possible to manage this complication with the insertion of a drain into the abdomen under CT guidance. This would be done by an interventional radiologist thus avoiding a trip to the operating room. However, it is sometimes necessary to perform an emergency operation because of a bowel perforation secondary to Avastin. While such perforations are unusual, one should always remember this possibility. I have treated a large number of patients with this drug and only one of them developed a bowel perforation.

The first patient to whom I gave Avastin was referred to me after failing several chemotherapy regimens. She presented with a CA 125 over 5,000 and a large, firm mass that extended from the left side of her rib cage down into the pelvis. The pressure produced by this mass obstructed the tube (ureter), which conveys urine from the kidney to the bladder. I was pleased to see that the mass disappeared and the CA 125 normalized after three months of treatment. She then developed the rare stroke-like syndrome associated with this drug, and although she recovered fully, I chose to stop the treatment.

In a very poignant moment in our relationship, she told me that if I stopped the drug she would die! I made a bargain with her. I told her that I would call the manufacturer, and if they would allow it, I would continue the treatment. The phone call was short and to the point. I was told that continuing this drug could produce a massive stroke transferring my patient to the vegetative state. Although she told me that she would accept that risk, I changed the treatment and she went on to die within the next six months.

I often think of what might have happened if I had continued treating her with Avastin. The work of the oncologist is more of a crap shoot than we would like to admit. Her response to this drug was nothing less than miraculous, and, had I continued it, the remission could have gone on for years and perhaps there would not have been any further neurologic complications. After all, she did tell me that she would take her chances, and that it was her life and her right to make such a decision. The *what ifs* and the *what might have beens* after a patient has died need to be placed in some sort of sealed bin or we would all go mad. Like so many other issues that oncologists must deal with, this was both a medical and an ethical dilemma.

By far the most interesting new group of drugs available for patients with ovarian cancer is the PARP inhibitors. These drugs inhibit the enzyme poly ADP ribose polymerase (PARP), which is an enzyme necessary in DNA repair. Chemotherapy may damage cancer cells without killing them. PARP is a protein that is important in the repair of single-stranded breaks in DNA, and so a PARP inhibitor will prevent the repair of the damaged cancer cell, thus hastening its death. Unlike chemotherapy drugs, which kill normal cells along with the cancer cells, these agents have the kindness to spare those normal cells that lack cancer-related alteration.

In patients with BRCA 1 or BRCA 2 mutations, PARP inhibitors cause multiple double strand breaks in DNA, leading us to believe that these drugs are more likely to be effective in patients with these genetic mutations. They have interesting names such as Iniparib, Olaparib, and Veliparib and are only available in a trial setting at this time. I was just informed that my practice was awarded a PARP inhibitor trial. Now I will not have to search all over the country for a place to send these very special patients.

PARP inhibitors are taken orally, have very few serious side effects, and have the potential to exert enormous benefit in patients with newly diagnosed and recurrent ovarian cancer. Unfortunately, I am not able to write a prescription for these pills as they are available only as part of investigational trials. Will they be helpful as an addition to chemotherapy regimens in common use either as first-line treatment or as treatment for a recurrence? If they are given after standard treatment has been completed (maintenance therapy), will they significantly diminish the chance for a recurrence? Will they produce a meaningful increase in the interval between the end of treatment and the appearance of a recurrence? This is the stuff of which dreams are made—a few pills a day and no recurrent tumor!

Because of the high risk of recurrent disease, the treating oncologist must never be led into a false sense of security. Once a remission lasts for several years the chance for a recurrence becomes almost geometrically less with each passing year, but it never becomes zero! When a patient has a recurrent ovarian cancer, a very important decision must be made with respect to the correct way to treat it. A recurrence is frequently located at the junction of the sigmoid colon and the rectum. If this is the only area seen on the CT scan then it would be appropriate to operate and remove that part of the colon, which is usually very easy to do. Almost all such patients will require chemotherapy postoperatively even though all visible cancer is removed.

If the imaging studies show widespread recurrent disease then all thought of surgery should be abandoned and chemotherapy started at once. Such patients have a much poorer prognosis than patients with an easily removable recurrence in a single area. Even those patients who have an excellent response to retreatment will have a high chance of developing another recurrence. What is needed is a method of mainte- nance therapy that has a low toxicity and can be given safely for many years.

8

THE FIRST SESSION

The river, spreading, flows—and spends your dream.
What are you, lost within this tideless spell?
—Hart Crane, *The Bridge*

I TRY TO be present in the chemotherapy suite when a new patient receives chemotherapy for the first time. Most people are far more frightened of this treatment than they are of surgery. The side effects are numerous and degrading and just about everybody has encountered a chemotherapy "horror show" in the person of a friend or family member. Even with all of the drugs that accompany the administration of chemotherapy, some of which impede consciousness, patients always seem to exit the suite at a much brisker pace than when they entered. One looks forward to surgery as a singular process. The process of chemotherapy is repetitive and carries with it intimations of mortality.

Several poignant stories have emerged from these encounters. One patient stared at the small suitcase that she brought with her and told me that the last time she packed it was for a trip to Paris. Another one looked dreamily into space and said, "This is my first time. You never forget your first!" I occasionally encounter gallows humor in the chemotherapy suite. Attempts at humor in this setting are mechanisms contrived to relieve stress and fear. The sight of others in neighboring chairs who have already received several courses of chemotherapy and who are sitting quietly eating potato chips and watching movies on television, exert a calming effect that no words from an oncologist could equal!

With the infusion of the first course of chemotherapy the patient has crossed the Rubicon, which of course, is a metaphor for not being able to turn back. It is not that the she can't choose to stop treatment after the first course; rather, almost all patients continue and finish the prescribed regimen. This is why it is so important for them to have confidence in their *team* and to feel comfortable in the environment in which the treatment is administered. This will be a long relationship, which hopefully will result in a cure. In a perfect setting the patient will look upon us as an extension of her family.

Rather than create a chapter that is distilled from bits of information from many different patients, I have decided to ask one woman to write this section for me. She had her first chemotherapy treatment last week and she composed this in an aura of confusion and disbelief, what I have come to call a state of luminous absence. Consciousness is at war with the desire to possess unconsciousness.

"I have lived with the diagnosis of ovarian cancer for a little over two weeks and I have seen three oncologists, and although I now have a plan that I can live with, everything remains surreal. I am not in my novel; I am in a Kafka novel! I always eat a healthy diet and I exercise almost every day and still this happened to me! It not only happened to me but Stage III happened to me. I was scheduled to have a chest port inserted on Friday, at 1:30 p.m. This was so hard for me, almost harder for me than the idea of chemotherapy. I could not picture myself with it sticking out of my chest wall, but I showed up on time and was ready to go. At the last minute one of the nurses came in to further explain what was about to happen to me. When I told her how frightened I was about the port she told me that Dr. Benigno always likes to have his patients remain in charge and she called him and he gave the OK for the port to be cancelled. I literally ran out of the radiology department.

"So here I am, walking slowly into the chemotherapy suite on Monday morning with my husband at my side. I am slightly out of my body. The part of me that is in my body, however, is trying to visualize bright, white light (brighter than those lights above me) flowing through me and healing me. I believe in the power of the mind. It is a wrestling match for sure. I guess that I am going to have to learn all the grips. The room is open and bright with huge windows all over the place. Everybody is polite and pleasant and they create such a welcoming environment. I would give anything to not need this welcome.

"When I signed in for the first chemotherapy session, a smiling, lovely nurse looked up at me from behind the glass and quickly ushered me back to the chemo suite. No matter what anybody tells you it is, of course, still your own experience. Yes, knowledge is king, and having preconceived ideas of what's to come is necessary and helpful, but this is my battle and no one else's. This is real and it is happening to me now. I am in the present tense! This transcends grammar. I so long for all of this to be in the past tense.

"Michael is my chemotherapy nurse and he introduces himself to me. He is calm and steady and I knew that this part was going to take a little time while we got to know one another. He showed me to a reclining chair with a window view and took my vital signs. I had my own television set but I knew that it would not provide any meaningful distraction during the first administration of chemotherapy.

"Michael looks at my veins and says, 'I see that you do not have a port. That is not a problem; you have great veins.' In two seconds he sticks me and gets into the vein on the first try, *in like Flynn*, and no pain! Michael explains everything about Carboplatinum and Taxol, the two chemotherapy drugs that I will be taking. He goes into everything, including the order and timing of administration and the side effects. He also told me about the medications that I would be taking for nausea, which made me feel a lot better because this was one of my biggest worries.

"Drip! Drip! Drip! Why does it take so long? I know that staring at the drops coming out of the infusion bag will not speed up the process but I just can't help it. I know that it is a poison. I know that it is also going to my good cells. Why is that? Why can't it go only to the cancer cells? I don't feel sick. I want to be any place but here, but now that I am here, I don't want to go through this anywhere else. I am going to have to stop confusing the issue!

"The session could not have been easier. I had snacks and soft drinks and my husband and sweet smiling nurses would come over and say hi and check on me. I didn't have any re-actions and was so grateful that the healing was beginning. During each drop that carried the chemotherapy from the IV bag into my body I imagined the explosion and death of large numbers of cancer cells. This is a battle that I intend to win!

"At home that evening I apparently heard a recording of a classical music recital but I have absolutely no recollection of this, so effective were the lingering effects of the anti-nausea medications. This is all so new to me. I took an Ambien and slept like a baby. I am less afraid than I was this morning but fear's chilling touch continues to hover over me. To have this day behind me is such a tremendous relief. My journey has begun."

Everything in such a scenario is important, especially what most people refer to as, "the little things." Let's get the big things out of the way first: She really does have ovarian cancer and needs chemotherapy; the drugs that she is getting are the correct drugs and are being administered in the appropriate dose; the nurses are trained in oncology and very experienced. These should be *givens* in every arena where chemotherapy is administered. Now for a discussion of those special things which are also very important to the healing process, little things that may not even invade the patient's consciousness!

One of the 20th century's most famous pianists once said that the art lies in the silences between the notes, something that is appreciated but difficult to define. With that in mind, let me talk about what some people call the small stuff. Is the staff professional at all times? Does the body language tell you that they would not want to be anywhere else at the moment other than helping you? Are conversations specific to you or are phrases recited out of a cookie cutter? Are you brought to your assigned chair immediately upon your arrival? Do you have the cell phone number of the chief chemotherapy nurse? The last item is of supreme importance as it tells you that everyone is really interested in your complete recovery and your return to a life unencumbered by what we are now doing to you. Sometimes what is not spoken carries with it the most important of all messages!

I have found that there is an enormous difference between the first and the second round of chemotherapy. Even though the hair is beginning to fall out and the bouts of nausea will be repetitive, the whole mess finally appears to be *doable*. Routine is everything in this scenario. Throughout subsequent treatments the prospect of recapturing one's previous life gradually unseats the specter of impending doom. Plans are made again. I have heard this thought expressed so often, "I never walk past a beautiful flower without slowing down. Nothing meaningful will ever be taken for granted again."

Perhaps even from cancer something good can emerge.

9

CLINICAL
TRIALS

Art is science made clear.

—Jean Cocteau

IF THERE EXISTED a perfect way to treat ovarian cancer, a treatment on which all clinicians could agree, there would be no need for clinical trials. A clinical trial investigates two or more treatment regimens for the same disease. Sometimes an experimental drug is included in the trial, one that has a *possible* but not a *proven* ability to make a positive difference. These are the trials that provide the oncologist with an ethical dilemma because it is possible that the experimental drug will produce poorer results than the established regimen. There has to be a very good reason to enter a patient into such a study and the informed consent document should reflect all of the downsides of the trial.

There are several types of clinical trials. It is of extreme importance that even the hint of bias be removed from the trial. This is best accomplished when the trial is randomized so that patients agree to a trial and are then assigned to one of the treatment arms by computer selection. Randomization takes away all possibility that an investigator can choose patients based on the possibility that they might do better with the study drug. A double-blind study occurs when neither the patient nor the clinician knows who is getting which drug. A prospective trial examines progress in an ongoing study whereas a retrospective study compares treatments by studying the medical records of patients.

The best studies are those which are both randomized and double blinded. The least scientific studies are ones that are retrospective. There are times when one of the study arms contains a placebo (no treatment). It has been my experience that studies that contain a placebo are the ones that are least likely to gain patient acceptance because they are afraid that if they do not get the study drug they will not do as well.

The proper running of a clinical trial setting is a very complicated process. Patients must be followed on a regular basis. Lab work and imaging studies must be ordered on a timely basis and record keeping must be perfect. The study must be presented to the patient completely and without bias of any kind. The study must be approved by a qualified institutional review board and a great deal of attention must be focused on the informed consent document. The clinical trial is where science meets ethics, and in such a situation ethics must always win.

It has been my experience that clinical trials do not work well when it is only the clinicians who are involved. It is absolutely necessary that a well-trained and experienced research nurse be appointed to supervise the trial. He or she is in charge of identifying possible candidates for the study, obtaining consent and randomization, collating all blood tests and imaging studies, and keeping perfect records. Without such a person, science suffers and the study could be fraught with error.

I am taking care of a patient at the present time whose cancer of the ovary recurred more than five years following surgery and chemotherapy. She is participating in a clinical trial, which requires retreatment with Carboplatinum and Taxol. The trial involves the possible administration of a study drug in addition to the chemotherapy. I am unable to tell her whether or not she is receiving the study drug because I simply do not know. I have the feeling that she thinks that I really do know the answer to this question and she has tried many different tricks to get the information out of me. It is very interesting that she is absolutely certain she is receiving the study drug because she feels "different" than she did the last time that she had chemotherapy.

Clinical trials are very important: They advance knowledge and help new treatments become part of established therapy; they have the potential, but *not* the certitude, that the outcome of the patients will improve because of the trial. A great deal of thought and soul-searching should go into the evaluation of a trial before it is approved and patients begin to accrue. I have one absolute rule: Is it a trial I would recommend to my wife or daughter? That question must be answered in the affirmative before consideration of the trial is allowed to go forward.

I had a very interesting experience recently. The practice was offered a clinical trial involving a new drug that was very difficult to obtain in this country. The trial had an enormous potential to help some of our patients. The drug would have been given to patients who developed a recurrent sarcoma of the uterus, an extremely rare and lethal disease. What made the study even more enticing was the fact that preliminary studies conducted in Europe showed great promise for this drug. There was one very unfortunate problem. They wanted us to treat the patients with a newly diagnosed sarcoma in a manner diametrically opposed to what we felt to be appropriate. If a recurrence were to occur, we would then be allowed to enter the patient into the trial. Needless to say, the offer was politely declined.

The following is a list of all the clinical trials for ovarian cancer currently available in my practice:

1. A Randomized, Open-Label Phase IIb Trial of Maintenance Therapy with a MUC1 Dendritic Cell Vaccine (CVac) for Epithelial Ovarian Cancer Patients in First or Second Remission

   (Can a vaccine made from the patient's white blood cells improve treatment results in recurrent disease?)

2. A Randomized, Double-Blinded, Placebo-Controlled Trial of Cvac (Autologous Dendritic Cells Pulsed with Recombinant Human Fusion Protein [Mucin 1-Glutathone S-Transferase] Coupled to Oxidized Polymerase as Maintenance Treatment in Patients with Epithelial Ovarian Cancer (EOC) in Complete Remission Following First-Line Chemotherapy

   (This study examines whether a vaccine given to newly diagnosed patients following standard chemotherapy can delay or prevent recurrent disease.)

3. A phase 2, Multi-Center, Double-Blind, Placebo Controlled, Randomized Study of Ombrabulin (a new vascular disruptive agent) in Patients with Platinum-Sensitive Recurrent Ovarian Cancer Treated with Carboplatinum/Paclitaxel

   (This study examines the effectiveness of a new vascular disruptive agent, which hopefully will be better and less toxic than Avastin.)

4. A Randomized Double-Blind Phase 3 Trial Comparing EC145 and Pegylated Liposomal Doxorubicin(PLD/ DOXIL /CAELYX) in Combination Versus PLD in Participants with Platinum-Resistant Ovarian Cancer

   (EC145 is Vinblastine chemotherapy with the addition of folic acid. We are trying to see if adding this to Doxil will improve survival in patients who have a recurrent cancer that was resistant to a platinum drug.)

5. A phase II Evaluation of the Poly(ADP-Ribose)-1 and-2 Inhibitor Velipanib (ABT-888) in the Treatment of Persistent or Recurrent Ovarian, Fallopian Tube or Primary Peritoneal Cancer in Patients who Carry a Germline BRCA 1 or BRCA 2 Mutation

    (This is a PARP inhibitor trial for patients who have recurrent ovarian cancer and who have a deleterious mutation on a BRCA gene.)

6. A Randomized Phase III Trial of Every-Three-Weeks Paclitaxel in Combination with Carboplatin with or without Concurrent and Consolidation Bevacizumab in the Treatment of Primary Stage III or IV Epithelial Ovarian, Peritoneal or Fallopian Tube Cancer

    (Will the addition of Bevacizumab (Avastin) improve survival in newly diagnosed advanced stage disease treated with standard chemotherapy?)

7. A Phase II Randomized Double-Blind Trial of Polyvalent Vaccine-KLH Conjugate (NSC 748933 IND#14384) + OPT-821 in Patients with Epithelial Ovarian, Fallopian Tube or Primary Peritoneal Cancer who are in Second or Third Complete Remission

    (This vaccine is combined with an immune booster [OPT-821] and given to patients who have been successfully treated for a first or second recurrence.)

8. A Phase II Clinical Trial of Bevacizumab (Avastin) with IV versus IP (intraperitoneal) Chemotherapy

in Ovarian, Fallopian Tube and Primary Peritoneal Cancer

(Will the addition of Bevacizumab (Avastin) to traditional chemotherapy improve survival in newly diagnosed patients treated with either intravenous or intraperitoneal platinum chemotherapy?)

9. Can Diet and Physical Activity Modulate Ovarian, Fallopian Tube and Primary Peritoneal Cancer Progress-Free Survival

10. Acquisition of Human Gynecologic Specimens to be used in Studying the Causes, Diagnosis, Prevention and Treatment of Cancer

Patients who are considering a clinical trial should investigate the trial thoroughly and examine the informed consent document very carefully. Not all clinical trials offer the same chance for an improvement in your condition and not all have the same propensity for side effects. It might help in the decision-making process for you to realize that all chemotherapy drugs in current usage were once part of a trial.

10

A DARK AND SAVAGE ROAD

Dark is a way and light is a place,
Heaven that never was
Nor will be ever is always true.
— Dylan Thomas, "Poem on His Birthday"

The median isn't the message.
— Stephen Jay Gould

We are all debts owed to death.
— Simonides of Ceos

A DARK AND savage road is a phrase that is borrowed from Robert Pinsky's magnificent translation of Dante's *Inferno*, and I can think of no better way to describe the experience of a patient undergoing chemotherapy for ovarian cancer. Among all of the many and varied duties of the oncologist is the obligation to transport the patient from an arena of darkness to a place of light! This cannot be accomplished in one visit. Constant attention to this issue on the part of the physician is mandatory, and the darkness begins to fade when the patient starts to believe that it is possible to put this mess behind her.

I have found that one of the best ways to assuage the anxieties and fears of the newly diagnosed patient is to put her in contact with patients who have made a similar journey many years ago, and who are doing well and are completely restored to a normal life as though nothing had ever happened. They exchange phone numbers and the previous patient acts as counselor and inspiration for the new patient. We schedule a large meeting of patients every quarter where women undergoing treatment meet and discuss numerous issues with survivors. There is no better way to help someone settle into this type of treatment routine. Many unusual friendships have emerged from this process and a number of patients have gathered together to form advocacy groups to lobby for funding, so that ovarian cancer research does not have to be breast cancer's poor sister.

The most extraordinary and prescient insight into a patient's reaction to the diagnosis of cancer is contained in the short essay "The Median Isn't the Message" by Stephen Jay Gould, the famous Harvard paleontologist, evolutionary biologist, and historian of science. It will be quoted widely now, for it is of the utmost use to oncologists and it is so comforting to patients that I frequently ask them to read it. At the age of 40, Dr. Gould developed an abdominal mesothelioma, a highly lethal form of cancer that took the life of the actor Steve McQueen.

After surgery he asked his oncologist to suggest some reading material and she told him that the medical literature contained nothing really worth reading, a ruse calculated to keep him away from the dreary statistics. Of course this remark speeded up his trip to the Harvard medical library and what he learned was profoundly depressing and frightening. What he did with this knowledge, however, offers a most important lesson for both oncologist and patient.

The terrifying statistic for this dreadful disease is that it carries with it a median survival of only eight months! Most people confuse the term median with mean or average. To arrive at the mean you simply add up all the survival data and then divide by the number of patients. The median, a measure of central tendency, is the half-way point. Stunned by the eight month statistic, Gould asked his friend Sir Peter Medawar, his scientific colleague and a Nobel Prize winner in immunology, what the best prescription for success against cancer might be. "A sanguine personality" was his terse reply, imbuing Gould with the very important message that attitude matters.

His initial thought that death was but eight months away became transposed to a belief that he would be among those who could live much longer, and he arrived at this conclusion through a process statisticians call *right skewed*. In a symmetrical distribution, the profile of variation to the left of the central tendency is a mirror image of variation to the right. In the skewed distribution related to abdominal mesothelioma, the variation to the right could stretch to sixty or seventy years, whereas the distribution to the left goes from eight months back to the day of diagnosis. Armed with the abundance of time that existed to the right of the central tendency, he could put on the back burner Isaiah's injunction to Hezekiah—"Set thine house in order: for thou shalt die, and not live" (Isaiah 38:1).

In his epic struggle with his own mortality, Gould pronounced death the ultimate enemy, and, in evaluating the swords of battle against his own demise, he found none more powerful than humor. When his death was announced at a meeting of paleontologists in Scotland he was reminded of Mark Twain's famous line: "The reports of my death are greatly exaggerated!" If humor is a sword in the battle against cancer then its absence arms the opposition.

Many years ago I encountered an oncologist who carried with him the aura of death. He would walk into a patient's room and announce the diagnosis. He would then tell the patient that he or she had a 95 percent chance of dying within the next eighteen months and would then make his exit after leaving a copy of the experimental protocol of which he was the principal investigator. Behavior of this kind produces anger and despair and it takes away from the patients all chance that they will arrive in the 5 percent survival bucket.

This is a good example of how statistics can harm and run counter to the healing process. Mark Twain, no great admirer of the medical profession, once said that there are three ways in which physicians contribute to the mendacity of society:

"There are lies, there are damn lies, and there are statistics!" In my opinion, candidates for medical school should be required to pass a mandatory test for a sense of humor!

11

DANA
REVISITED

Like the experience of warfare, the endurance of grave or terminal illness involves long periods of tedium and anxiety, punctuated by briefer interludes of stark terror and pain.

—Christopher Hitchens

Vanish.
Pass into nothingness: the Keats line that frightened her.

—Joan Didion

I'm not afraid to die. I just don't want to be there when it happens.

—Woody Allen

THERE ARE MANY cancers in which a five-year survival is meaningful, a cause for celebration. One can allow the horrific memories of surgery and chemotherapy to be placed on life's back burner and have reason to believe that there will not be a recurrence. Although the memory of that savage road will never be effaced completely, the fifth anniversary places a barrier between the patient and all thought of a recurrence. Not so with epithelial ovarian cancer. The train always seems to be in the dark tunnel, about to emerge at full speed at the shrill whistle of a positive CT scan.

Thirteen years after Dana's last chemotherapy treatment she came into my office earlier than her scheduled appointment complaining of abdominal pain and bloating. I remember saying to myself that it can't be a recurrent cancer. It had been well over ten years since all treatment had been stopped. My experience, however, told me otherwise. After all, the symptoms were the same as they were when she was newly diagnosed.

Dana was frightened and had a faraway look in her eyes that oncologists see so often, a look that announces the appearance of a recurrence even before the diagnosis is confirmed. The CT scan revealed a pelvic mass which in her case could only mean that the cancer had returned. When I discussed the findings with her she asked me in a calm, monotone voice if this meant that she would need more surgery and chemotherapy and my affirmative answer was met with an expletive that I am told airline pilots scream out shortly before the plane goes down.

Dana underwent a second operation and the recurrence was found in the recto-sigmoid colon, necessitating the removal of that part of the colon. The remaining colon was stapled together, interdicting the need for a colostomy. Chemotherapy was restarted soon after the operation and, because of the advent of newer and more effective anti-nausea medications, was much better tolerated than the initial treatment. Several years later, she developed another recurrence. There ensued a waltz that oncologists witness all too frequently; changes in chemotherapy producing shorter and shorter remissions.

Dana was eventually treated with a combination of Avastin and Abraxane, which is a newer form of Taxol. The treatment/remission scenario was played out for a number of years during which she led a fairly normal life except, of course, for the chemotherapy sessions. She was able to work, was usually free of pain, and went on holidays with her husband.

At the end of another remission a repeat CT scan showed a mass in the pelvis and some nodularity in the upper abdomen. I had a long talk with Dana and told her that additional chemotherapy had no chance of getting rid of the tumor. I had stopped using the word cure, a fact that did not go unnoticed. I discussed with her the option of yet another surgical procedure that almost certainly would involve a colon resection with the strong possibility that she might require a permanent colostomy. I was concerned that this would be a bridge too far and I was also worried that because of the extraordinary length of time that I had worked with her it might be possible that my emotional attachment to this great lady might be impeding my clinical judgment. I insisted that she get another opinion and I sent her to Paul Sabattini, who heads the ovarian cancer division at Sloan Kettering in New York City. She returned to Atlanta with a green light for the surgery.

Some twenty-three years after her original diagnosis Dana underwent yet another surgical procedure with the findings of extensive tumor involving the rectum as well as multiple nodules around several loops of small intestine. Most of the rectum was removed and three separate small bowel resections were performed, thus removing all visible tumor. The bowel was put together and no colostomy was necessary. She tolerated this extensive surgery without difficulty and was discharged within a week. Each morning on rounds I would marvel at the courage of this very brave lady who had lived under the Sword of Damocles for almost a quarter of a century.

When cancer of the ovary recurs after such extensive surgery and chemotherapy, it tends to produce an even greater darkness and fear than that which accompanied the initial diagnosis. The patient feels betrayed by her own expectations. However, this time she knows the drill only too well. It is the beginning of the second act and the action involves more chemotherapy with its attendant nausea and hair loss and possibly another trip to the operating room. Even people who have never prayed before mumble a few words asking that this dreadful play be assigned but two acts and that the curtain never rises again to usher in yet another recurrence. There ensues a rage, the darkest rage, lightened by nothing. No matter how large and loving the family, a feeling of isolation and dissociation pervades all aspects of her life. Loneliness and aloneness become part of the daily routine. As Stéphane Mallarmé so eloquently wrote, she is riding the "indeterminate wave in which all reality dissolves."

12

THE
RECURRENCE

As if the normal above-water state of things, the sober delimitation of our existence, were but a brief parenthesis overwhelmed in an instant.

—Roberto Calasso
The Marriage of Cadmus and Harmony

THIS WILL BE a short and a rather uplifting chapter. I selected this patient to serve as a smashing rebuttal to all of the entries on the Internet that say, in no uncertain terms, that a recurrent cancer of the ovary is a death sentence that is carried out rather quickly. I did not want the reader to think that the Dana's thirteen-year progression-free survival was a very great rarity.

Carla is a truly unique patient in many ways. *The Sword of Damocles* is a metaphor for impending doom and I have mentioned how most patients who have been diagnosed with ovarian cancer feel such an object suspended above them even if they have never heard of the Greek legend. In Carla's case there was not even a walnut above her head. She took neither her disease nor me seriously, and that, I am certain, has contributed greatly to her extraordinary outcome. She never complained and even my finely honed perspicacity was unable to detect those common emotions such as fear or anger.

I met her in 1998 when her abdomen was stacked to the top with ovarian cancer. I gave her several rounds of chemotherapy and then operated on her and removed all of the cancer. I think that it will be more helpful if I summarize the course of her treatment in several terse statements:

- 1998—Treatment begins
- Three courses of chemotherapy with Carboplatinum and Taxol
- Extensive surgery
- Six additional courses of chemotherapy with Carboplatinum and Taxol
- Extensive surgery for recurrent disease
- Twelve courses of Doxil chemotherapy
- Several other recurrences treated with Gemzar followed by Topotecan and then Carboplatinum again
- Completed 34 courses of bi-weekly Taxol
- Refused additional chemotherapy
- Oral Megace (Progesterone hormone) 2004 to the present
- CA 125 drops precipitously
- CT scan shows no evidence of disease in 2010

- 2011—CA 125 begins to rise
- CT scan shows minimal recurrent disease in the pelvis
- Refuses chemotherapy again
- Repeat CT scan in November 2012 (six months later) shows very minimal progression

An hour before I wrote this paragraph she was presented to the weekly tumor board meeting and nine oncologists had the opportunity to review her remarkable history. No one was very enthusiastic about restarting chemotherapy, although I will review this option with her more out of duty than passion. She is truly above it all, existing in her own world and managing all aspects of her life including the medical decisions. She reminds me of the famous Frank Sinatra song, "I did it my way."

Carla is one of my favorite patients, but I cannot help but feel that she sometimes considers me an annoying intrusion into an otherwise peaceful life. She occasionally turns down one of my therapeutic recommendations with the flippant remark, "I don't have time for this; I'm going on a cruise!" As you might imagine, she is a wonderful help to those patients who have a newly diagnosed recurrent cancer. She will not cancel a cruise for me, but once on dry land she is always there to lend a helping hand and a warm heart.

It is now almost sixteen years since her original diagnosis of advanced cancer of the ovary. During most of this time she has been taking a few progesterone hormone pills each day and on numerous occasions has refused my furtive recommendations that she revisit chemotherapy. As of the writing of this paragraph she is planning her next cruise! Where is it written that the oncologist, and not the patient, has all the right answers? Please remember that all gynecologic oncologists have such patients!

13

JOHN MCDONALD

His life was gentle; and the elements
So mix'd in him that Nature might stand up
And say to all the world, this was a man!

—William Shakespeare
Julius Caesar, Act V

He is a system of northern lights, an aurora borealis
visible where most of us will never go.

—Harold Bloom
Shakespeare: The Invention of the Human

THERE ARE SOME men who defy description. How can someone of such genius be so self-effacing? I have worked with John McDonald for more than twelve years and, without fanfare of any kind, the work is done perfectly and with a level of integrity and attention to detail that is truly remarkable. He attends board meetings in jeans, rides a motorcycle, and is able to captivate a disparate audience with a combination of brilliance and charm. In addition to his scientific skills, he is able to bring together researchers from many different departments at Georgia Tech, including nanotechnology, bioinformatics, and bioengineering, and convince them to participate in our research efforts. This is a gift totally unrelated to scientific prowess.

He began his alliance with the Ovarian Cancer Institute as its chief research scientist twelve years ago. He holds an undergraduate degree in philosophy and biology and earned a PhD in genetics at the University of California, Davis. He has an outstanding reputation for research to which his four books and 141 articles published in peer review journals would attest. He began his career with the Institute while he was a professor and department head of genetics at the University of Georgia. To my everlasting delight he was appointed chair of the School of Biology at the Georgia Institute of Technology. The University put a considerable sum of money into our research laboratories and we were at last up and running. When John realized that almost all of his research involved the serum and tissue samples sent to him from my operating room, he resigned as chair of biology to devote himself full time to our research.

Early in our relationship John became quite enamored of the quality of the tissue samples that he was receiving because they were so pristinely collected and flash-frozen within ten seconds of their removal from the patient. All reviewers of our publications have commented on how perfect the DNA was. Not only is the tissue and serum banked but the entire patient history as well as follow-up data are entered into a computerized data bank, which is one of the largest such data banks for ovarian cancer in the world. The ongoing research projects that the Ovarian Cancer Institute is conducting at the McDonald Laboratory in the School of Biology at the Georgia Institute of Technology are summarized as follows:

1. **Ovarian Cancer Stem Cell Project.** Cancer stem cells or cancer initiating cells are believed to be the origin of all cancers. These stem cells typically are contained within tumors in low frequency (it has been estimated that less than 1 percent of the cancer cells making up a tumor are cancer stem cells). Unlike the bulk of cancer cells making up a tumor, cancer stem cells do not replicate rapidly. Most traditional chemotherapy drugs have been selected for use because they attack rapidly dividing cells. These drugs often attack and kill the majority of the cancer cells but they do not kill the cancer stem cells. This may explain why ovarian cancer has such a high recurrence rate. Our researchers have been able to isolate ovarian cancer stem cells from both ovarian cancer cell lines as well as from ovarian cancer cells present in ascites, which is the fluid in the abdomen produced from the cancer.

   Over the past year, we have shown that ovarian cancer stem cells are not effectively killed by the drugs commonly used in the treatment of ovarian cancer. We are currently developing new therapies that can either directly kill ovarian cancer stem cells or stimulate these stem cells to be converted to the type of cancer cells that can be killed by conventional types of therapy.

2. **Personalized Cancer Therapy Project.** The traditional approach to cancer chemotherapy consists of finding a drug that effectively arrests cancer cells grown in laboratory culture conditions. Promising drugs are then tested in laboratory animal models. If a drug passes these tests, it moves to a phase one experimental trial in humans. The effectiveness of an experimental drug in humans is determined by monitoring how well it does in reducing tumor growth in the majority of patients tested. Many drugs that work dramatically in a few patients but not in the majority of patients are discarded and not granted FDA approval for general use.

We now realize that this approach is flawed because cancer is not one single disease. We desperately need to find a way to identify the small cohort of patients who will respond to the uncommon drugs as these are the very people who will fail the regimen which works for the majority of patients. There is extensive genetic variation even among the same family of cancers and between specific cancer patients. This means that not only can cancer progress differently in different patients but these patients may respond differently to the same cancer drug. The promise of a personalized approach to drug therapy is based on our current ability to genetically categorize each patient's tumor on the molecular level. By analyzing each patient's tumor individually, we are developing computational methods to identify the most appropriate chemotherapy for each individual patient.

3. The Use of Nanoparticles in the Treatment of Ovarian Cancer: Targeted Drug Delivery with Nanohydrogels.

Nanohydrogels are nanoparticles that we use to carry therapeutic RNA into cancer cells. Current chemotherapy is focused on compounds that inhibit or otherwise block the function of proteins that are aberrantly expressed in cancer cells. This approach is inherently limited for two reasons: First, it has been estimated that less than 10 percent of all human genes are even potentially *drugable* at the protein level; second, the levels of protein inhibiting drugs needed to kill all of the cancer cells cannot be tolerated by most patients. One possible solution to this problem is to inhibit aberrant gene expression at the RNA level rather than at the protein level. Unlike protein inhibitors, antagonistic RNA (RNA that has the capacity to combat cancer RNA) has the potential to inhibit any gene in the human genome. We know that this approach to cancer therapy works amazingly well when tested in cancer cell cultures. The problem occurs when we try to target these inhibitory molecules specifically to cancer cells without affecting the healthy cells.

In collaboration with Dr. Andrew Lyon in the School of Chemistry and Biochemistry at Georgia Tech, we are using nanohydrogel spheres that can be filled with chemotherapy drugs that specifically target ovarian cancer cells. We have published a series of papers demonstrating the utility of this method of targeted drug delivery to ovarian cancer cells grown in culture. We have recently received funding from the National Institutes of Health (NIH) to demonstrate the usefulness of this method in mouse model systems. Such animal studies are a necessary prelude to the introduction of this novel technology to phase one human trials.

4. **The Use of Nanoparticles in the Treatment of Ovarian Cancer: The Magnetic Nanoparticle Project.** Most ovarian cancer metastases are caused by cancer cells sloughing off the primary tumor into the abdominal cavity and spreading to the omentum, the capsule of the liver, and other peritoneal surfaces. In collaboration with Dr. John Zhang in the School of Chemistry at Georgia Tech, Dr. John Mcdonald and Dr. Ken Scarberry have constructed magnetic nanoparticles that can be specifically targeted to ovarian cancer cells. We have recently shown that these nanoparticles can be incorporated into a perfusion system (similar to a dialysis system) and used outside the body to capture and isolate the cancer cells in a mouse model system. Our success in developing this novel technology has captured the interest of the biotechnology industry.

Work on all four of these projects is continuing at a fervent and rapid pace and is hindered only by the problems encountered in raising money in these difficult and uncertain times. The cultivation of stem or progenitor cells is of extreme importance because it is these cells that survive standard chemotherapy. It is easy to kill off the daughter cells with such treatment but the stem cells, which comprise less than 1 percent of the total cell population in ovarian cancer, are resistant to chemotherapy and are responsible for the extremely high recurrence rate.

We have recently identified a panel of drugs that will kill ovarian cancer stem cells in cell culture. If these results are validated in animal models, they can be tested in phase one human trials. We are hopeful that this new spectrum of anti-stem cell drugs will be of value not only in ovarian cancer but also in the entire spectrum of cancer because all cancers have stem cells!

Major breakthroughs in such work will not necessarily come from famous and extremely well-funded research centers. We need to remember that Sir Alexander Fleming discovered penicillin by accident while working alone in a decrepit laboratory and that Sidney Farber directed the development of Aminopterin for the treatment of childhood leukemia while working in a small, badly heated basement room.

14

THE TEST—
FURTHER
INROADS

History is that certainty produced at the point where the imperfections of memory meet the inadequacies of documentation.

—Julian Barnes
The Sense of an Ending

TWELVE YEARS HAVE gone by and more than 2,000 tissue and serum samples have been sent to the Ovarian Cancer Institute for analysis. These include not only samples from patients with ovarian cancer but also samples from patients with benign tumors as well as those with normal ovaries. All patients signed a consent form for this analysis and were told that genetic testing would be done. Only two patients refused to participate, an indication of the strong desire of these women to see a viable and highly accurate screening test discovered as soon as possible. After all, there was no experimentation on them; only on the tissue that was going to be removed anyway.

The process must be as seamless as it is accurate because a single error in the identification of a patient can make a meaningful difference in the analysis of the data. The serum, tissue, and data must be handled perfectly and stored properly or the material is useless for study. It is very important that a well-qualified person be in charge of these delicate issues— someone who shares with the surgeon and chief research scientist a passion for accuracy and a commitment to excellent results. The Ovarian Cancer Institute is lucky to have such a tireless worker in the person of Kim Toten, who stands behind me in the operating room with an open canister of liquid nitrogen so that the tissue removed from the patient can be immediately flash-frozen, thus preserving forever the viability of the tissue for future study. Her duties also include the storage of the patient data as well as the transfer of tissue and serum to the large minus 80 degree Celsius freezer at Georgia Tech. She was formerly an operating room nurse at my hospital and I stole her for the Institute—all is fair in love and war!

Using the microarray analyzer, we were able to identify genes that are aberrantly expressed in ovarian cancer tissue. This information is very useful in understanding the molecular basis of the cancer in individual patients and in the design of personalized therapies. However, any potential screening test for ovarian cancer will not be based on the analysis of tissue. Screening tests need to be minimally invasive and thus are limited to the use of easily collected body fluids (blood, urine, etc.) for their analysis.

The Ovarian Cancer Institute has taken a novel approach to the development of an accurate screening test for ovarian cancer. Rather than looking for the abnormal expression of one or a few proteins in blood (such as the CA 125 biomarker for ovarian cancer or the PSA test for prostate cancer, neither of which is sufficiently accurate), we decided to look for diagnostic differences in the levels of metabolites circulating in the blood. Metabolites are the products of cellular reactions that go on in our cells and can be indicative of molecular level changes that occur at very early stages of cancer development.

Several years ago we initiated studies looking for differences in metabolic patterns in blood sera collected from ovarian cancer patients versus blood sera collected from normal, healthy women. These initial studies were carried out by mass spectrometry (MS) in collaboration with Dr. Facundo Fernandez in the School of Chemistry at Georgia Tech. A mass spectrometer is a complicated instrument that can determine the relative levels of thousands of metabolites in the blood.

Because the data generated from such MS analyses are massive and extremely complicated, we recruited Dr. Alex Gray from the College of Computer Science at Georgia Tech. Dr. Gray is an expert in pattern recognition algorithms. Much to our delight, we found that there is indeed a clear metabolic pattern that is diagnostic of ovarian cancer. Moreover, the pattern is highly accurate in distinguishing sera collected from ovarian cancer patients relative to sera collected from normal healthy controls.

The results of our initial study were published in 2010 in the journal *Cancer Epidemiology, Biomarkers and Prevention*. We found that in forty-four women with serous papillary carcinoma of the ovary and fifty women with benign conditions, our assay was able to distinguish between cancer and control groups with an unprecedented accuracy (100 percent sensitivity and 98 percent specificity). We classified one woman in our control group as having cancer whose tumor was actually benign. However, since this woman came from a family with a long history of ovarian cancer (both her mother *and* grandmother had died of ovarian cancer), we felt it was possible that our test may have detected a very early manifestation of this disease. This individual continues to be monitored very closely.

What wonderful news! We had an assay that could detect ovarian cancer with 100 percent accuracy. What a contrast to the CA 125 test, which is negative in 20 percent of those women who have ovarian cancer! Much to my dismay, John McDonald was guarded in his enthusiasm. He felt that we had to validate that the test was equally as accurate in women with Stage I cancers. Since the few early stage samples included in our initial study were also correctly classified, he remains confident that the assay will prove to be accurate when we are able to test a large number of samples from patients with early stage disease. Serum samples from patients with Stage I ovarian cancer are extremely rare and we had to purchase, at considerable expense, thirty of these samples from around the world. Nobody wants a diagnostic test that becomes positive only in patients with advanced stage disease.

But John pointed out another difficulty. While our initial results were tremendously exciting, the metabolic patterns we identified were just that; patterns, or in the lingo of mass spectrometry chemists, mass-charge ratios. Thus, although we knew that metabolic changes in sera are extremely accurate in diagnosing ovarian cancer (a major breakthrough in its own right), we did not know the identity of the specific metabolic molecules that were indicative of this disease. Without this specific information the assay would likely not be able to acquire FDA approval and not be of interest to the industrial sector for commercial development. This was very hard for me to comprehend and I still find it shocking. No commercialization, no test! The completion of this work would take longer than I had anticipated. John told me that I would have to wait.

I became somewhat agitated! What do you mean, I have to wait? I am a surgeon with a type A personality. I want definitive answers yesterday! I was unable to get anything else out of him. I would have to put up with what might turn out to be a long series of delays, and patience is hardly one of my virtues. However, if one of us needs to approach this work in a cold and unemotional manner I guess it should be the scientist. There is no room for wishful thinking which might lead to error. I want this test to be 100 percent accurate more than anything else that I have ever wanted in my career and

John McDonald is around to remove fantasy and distill results from raw data.

The smoke has finally settled, revealing two diametrically opposed people. John McDonald would be as lost in the operating room as I would be in a basic science laboratory. It became obvious that we were far from being able to move forward with a widely available diagnostic test. Too much time had elapsed from the original publication in 2010, an interval that saw the arrival of a new mass spectrometer which would require its own set of calibrations and, as if that were not bad enough, there were new post-doctoral fellows working on the machine.

The first order of the day was to determine the identity of our diagnostic patterns and then validate the assay on our recently acquired Stage I samples. I saw *time's winged chariot* drawing near and there was nothing that I could do about it. There are some things that a scalpel cannot fix!

15

IN THEIR OWN WORDS

Perhaps the whole course of a human life is merely a narrative created to make sense to our weak intellects of a dozen or so really powerful dreams.

—Sigmund Freud

THIS INTERESTING QUOTATION from Freud was chosen because in listening to patients recount their innermost emotions when they receive the diagnosis of cancer and begin therapy, the one almost universal thread is that it is a dreamlike state. *"This is not happening to me!"* A feeling of detached imagination produces a faraway look that is not so much fear as it is a suspension of reality. Therapists can be of great help in a patient's adjustment not only to the diagnosis but also to all of the ramifications that surround the onset of treatment. However, I have found that ultimately it is the treating physician and his or her staff who provide the major support system and eventually serve as a bulkhead against the forces of fear and the sense of impending doom.

It is important that the patient return to her everyday routine as soon as possible. The worst scenario is the fetal position in bed in a constant state of worry and turmoil. I ask my patients to outline four fifteen-minute periods a day when they are allowed to dwell on these problems— 8:00–8:15— 12:00–12:15, and so on. This helps to "compartmentalize" the fear and agony and allows for a much more normal lifestyle. If these emotions rear their ugly heads at 10:00 in the morning, they are asked to look at their watches and say out loud, "It's not time now; I will think about this later." As silly as this appears, it actually works. Nomenclature has its uses and in these situations not even cancer should be nameless and unspeakable. After all, it is what it is. Listen to it, pronounce it another six letter word and move on. *March forward into the past tense!*

The importance of routine in desperate situations is eloquently brought home in a poem by Rudyard Kipling:

> *Hearts may fail, and Strength outwear, and Purpose*
>   *turn to Loathing,*
> *But the everyday affair of business, meals, and clothing,*
> *Builds the bulkhead 'twixt Despair and the Edge of*
> *Nothing.*

I have never encountered a more powerful statement addressing the value of returning to an everyday routine as a method of dealing with disaster. Neither patient nor physician is a stranger to despair. The trick is to avoid the precipice that leads to the edge of nothing, and an adherence to a routine is the best way to accomplish this. Get up at the same time each morning, have a cup of coffee and read the newspaper. Each day needs to have a plan.

T.S. Eliot gave the best definition ever of the dance. *"At the still point of the turning world. Neither flesh nor fleshless;Neither from nor towards; at the still point, there the dance is."* I respectfully suggest that cancer is the still point of the turning life. Everything comes to a crashing halt and an eerie stillness pervades all aspects of one's being. It is a wake without death and it imparts to the recipient a feeling of isolation and *otherworldliness* that never completely goes away.

I have asked several of my patients to write down a personal memoir of their experiences from the moment that they received the diagnosis of ovarian cancer until the moment they took pen to hand. What emerged was a set of documents at the same time unique and universal. Their stories have helped me in immeasurable ways to understand cancer through the optic of a personal journey, and, in so doing, they have made me a better doctor.

CATHERINE'S STORY

At my request Catherine wrote down her thoughts surrounding her illness. It is such a remarkable document that I will recount it in its entirety.

Is Something Wrong?

"I guess it all started in January of last year. My husband and I were in a happy place. We'd been married just over a year and our careers were skyrocketing. We loved our lives; we had two great dogs and enough income to travel once or twice a year. We had no plans to have children; instead our dream was to adopt an older child or two in our 40s. I was 37 years old and working as an IT manager at a large company when I started noticing that I just didn't feel right. I felt "gassy" and bloated all the time. At first I thought it was the birth control pill that I was on so I had my doctor put me on a lower dose pill. After another month I went back to my doctor to let him know I still felt "thick and gassy" all the time. He then started testing me for gastrointestinal problems and had me get an abdominal and transvaginal ultrasound. The ultrasound showed a small cyst on my right ovary, but the doctor said not to worry. All women have cysts on their ovaries as part of the menstrual cycle and he went on to say that he would check it again in six weeks.

OK, Now I Know Something's Wrong!

"The last week in March I flew to San Francisco from Atlanta and when I stood up to get off the plane there was a horrible pain in my left groin area. It felt like I was trying to rip a muscle in two. As I walked off the plane, it seemed to lessen a bit and I was able to make it to the car with the rest of the group I was traveling with. During the whole four days in San

Francisco I was scared that I was going to have to go to the emergency room while on a business trip. How embarrassing would that be? Every time I stood up I would have the horrible pain and have to walk it off for several minutes.

"While I was still in San Francisco I emailed my doctor and made an appointment for the day I got home. He sent me straight to the hospital to have an emergency CT scan. That was Friday morning. Friday afternoon the nurse called me and asked if I could return to the office on Monday morning. I knew it was something bad. My husband and I went to see my doctor on Monday morning and he told me that I had four cysts and that it could be either endometriosis or cancer. CANCER!?! I could not have cancer. There is no way I have cancer.

My Angels!

"The next day I went to see Dr. Benigno, who is a gynecologic oncologist. He reviewed my scans and ordered some more tests. My CA125 came back and it was 91, not terribly high, but higher than normal. At first I freaked out but the nurse told me the test had a huge false positive percentage, which helped me to worry just a little bit less. So the doctor scheduled surgery for April 5. If it is endometriosis then it would be just a simple laparoscopic surgery. If it is something else, well, let's just wait and see. I told Dr. Benigno that if the easiest and best solution was to take it all out then just do it. It's going to be endometriosis anyway, right? I made a deal with my husband, the first words out of his mouth after surgery had to be, "You don't have cancer." I didn't realize that I was asking him to do something so hard. After the surgery I was being taken to my room and I saw him and my friend with the most heartbreaking looks on their faces. I asked him, "Is it cancer?" and he replied, "I think that you already know it is." My world went black.

"The next memory that I have is waking up in my hospital room with my husband next to me and Dr. Benigno and his nurse Sherry standing at the foot of the bed. Dr. Benigno apologized to me and said that he didn't really think it was going to be cancer and then I asked if I was going to die. He emphasized that all of the cancer was removed and that I would need to have chemotherapy. He told me that with ovarian cancer no one could predict outcome. In addition to the removal of my uterus, tubes, and ovaries the appendix, omentum, and part of my bowel were removed. I had a Stage III C ovarian cancer.

"Dr. Benigno encouraged me to make plans to do something special on the first anniversary of the surgical procedure so that I would have something fun to look forward to. My husband went home that night and made reservations at a world famous restaurant for April 5 of the following year. We now had something to look forward to that would be fun!

The Fight Begins!

"I had a twelve-inch vertical incision on my abdomen and two smaller incisions on each side with a total of fifty-seven staples. I could not sit up without using my arms for weeks and it took almost two weeks before I had a bowel movement or could get through a night without a heavy dose of pain killers. My family came to town and stayed with us for a few weeks and neighbors and friends brought me food and anything else I needed. I then began chemotherapy with Carboplatinum and Taxol.

"I was feeling pretty spunky up to this point. This was something I could beat; I am a strong person. Well, chemotherapy is stronger! I was stupid and didn't call Dr. Benigno or the nurses even though I had their personal cell phone numbers. The first few days after the chemotherapy were unbelievably difficult with profound nausea and vomiting. I couldn't move, eat, drink, or sleep.

"I went to the emergency room and they gave me Zofran and Phenergan but I still threw up an hour later. Finally, six days after the treatment I let them know that I was in really bad shape and I returned to the infusion center for intravenous fluids. That's all it took and I felt so much more human! It turned out that the regular anti-nausea drugs don't work very well for me and once they were changed, subsequent chemotherapy treatments became much easier.

"I lost my hair within the first fourteen days and my eyebrows and eyelashes after the fifth cycle of treatment. My veins stopped cooperating around the third cycle, necessitating the insertion of an intravenous chest port for the rest of the treatments. I am now finished with all chemotherapy, my CT scan is negative and my CA125 is three.

Looking Back!

"In hindsight I see that I really did have the symptoms of ovarian cancer in the beginning. I was so frustrated by my weight. No matter how much I worked out or how little I ate I kept gaining weight around my middle. I went from a size 6 to a 14 in just two years even though my diet and exercise routine improved. After the surgery my belly was normal. I had never thought to tell my doctor about the weight gain. I just thought that I was getting old and fat. As part of my care, I was genetically tested and learned that I am BRCA 1 positive which means that I have a higher risk of developing breast cancer and so now I have to think about that also.

"Being grateful has a new meaning for me now. I have two doctors who saved my life: One who took my ambiguous symptoms seriously and the other who took out all of the cancer and who knew the best way to treat it. I have a boss who did my job and his during the six months I was out and I have friends and neighbors who kept my spirits up and brought me food, flowers, or sometimes just a laugh. I have a family who dropped everything to be with me when I needed them.

What Next?

"I have no idea. Maybe the cancer comes back and maybe it doesn't. I need to learn to live with that and be grateful for every day."

I have never encountered a more complete or more poignant recounting of a woman's awakening to the fear and reality of ovarian cancer. It is the very apotheosis of the epic struggle peculiar to all patients with this disease. Last month there was a fashion show put on by Tootsie's, a high end clothing store in Atlanta, which benefited the Ovarian Cancer Institute. When Catherine had just finished with her chemotherapy treatments she was one of the models at the event. She walked down the runway engulfed in a stunning luminosity, proving to all around her that even ovarian cancer can be put in its place!

ANITA

This patient was in her early 60s and recently married for the first time when the unthinkable happened. The symptoms were loud and clear and roared rather than whispered. She sat in my office with her husband, and, even though she was well aware of the results of the CT scan, she did not believe it until she heard it from me. Vocabulary is everything in these situations. Words can heal as well as destroy. I asked her to tell me what was wrong with her.

"It all began about a year ago when I was having gastro-intestinal problems. Going to one of the top GI specialists in Atlanta I thought my problem would soon be solved. I had this feeling of bloating which actually got better for awhile until it came back with a vengeance. It seems that I had a different test each month until a CT scan was finally done and I heard the word *cancer*. I was in a state of shock and disbelief. How did this happen? There was no cancer in my family and the last physical exam that I had was perfectly normal."

This is all too common. Anita had symptoms for almost a year before the diagnosis was made and at the time of surgery there was so much cancer in the abdomen that in addition to removing the uterus, tubes, and ovaries, 90 percent of the colon as well as the spleen needed to be removed. She was treated with Carboplatinum and Taxol and has developed recurrences requiring changes in chemotherapy. She has had Doxil and, after that, Topotecan. Each time that the chemotherapy is changed the news is greeted with an equanimity that I find astonishing. Far from allowing this process to take over her life, she travels frequently and recently was able to go to Europe for an extended holiday.

Throughout all of the jousting with the cancer and using all sorts of chemotherapy drugs, Anita does not appear ill. She looks good and leads a normal life except for the treatment sessions. Unfortunately, there is no way to predict which chemotherapy drugs will be the most effective for an individual patient at a given time in her treatment process. The first-line treatment always includes Carboplatinum and Taxol, but there is an unacceptable level of resistance to these drugs as well as a high recurrence rate. The management of a platinum resistant ovarian cancer is one of our most daunting challenges. To make matters worse, when the cancer comes back there is still no unanimity of opinion in the oncology community with regard to the best way to treat these patients.

Anita has been told that with the currently available modalities of treatment little likelihood exists that all of the tumor will disappear. The struggle involves reducing what is unfortunately called the "tumor burden" so that she reaches a homeostasis with the cancer. A *Wild West* standoff exists in that I am not able to harm the cancer further and the cancer is not able to harm my patient. This is not a very comforting state of existence, but it is one that is not only accepted but also actually sought after in situations such as this. My patients frequently tell me that this condition is better than the alternative!

JEAN

"My doctor will not return my telephone calls; I have an advanced cancer of the ovary and I don't know what is happening to me. I am being treated with chemotherapy and I don't seem to have a plan. What is going on? I know that I am 80 years old but I don't feel like dying right now. Dr. Benigno, I can't think of anything else except this God-awful problem. I used to have many interests but now ovarian cancer is at the center stage of my life. I want you to put this cancer on the back burner, preferably my husband's back burner!"

No one had ever suggested that I transpose a cancer to someone else's back burner much less the backburner of the husband! I found that request as draconian as it was unusual, but since the South is a matriarchy, I felt that the only appropriate reply was "Yes Ma'am." This request induced in me a quasi moral conundrum. What if I actually had the ability to transpose a cancer in one of my patients to someone else? Hopefully, by now the reader will believe that I would never even think of such a thing. However, the morality of such an issue would make an interesting topic in a course on medical ethics.

This patient transferred her care to my practice in the middle of neo-adjuvant chemotherapy (chemotherapy administered before surgery) for an advanced cancer of the ovary. She was confused and frightened and needed the input of many members of the team to finally assuage her anxieties. This is a very good example of the value of communication as a weapon in the armory of the oncologist. Repetitive discussions with one's oncologist serve to take away darkness, and, where cancer is concerned, we are all afraid of the dark.

I operated on her and it was very easy to remove the tumor. At the age of 80 she withstood several hours of surgery without difficulty and her recovery was uneventful. She was very easy to take care of once all of her questions were answered and she understood the treatment that was recommended.

Following her surgery she completed her chemotherapy and continues to do well. She rarely comes to the office without the gift of a book or a Bach recording.

JUDY

"There was a time, not very long ago at all, that I did not know how (or if) I'd ever be able to get out of bed again. So to be here today, sharing my story, feels much like a dream. I was 38 years old when I was diagnosed with Stage III cancer of the ovary and I am a textbook example of how difficult this disease is to diagnose and treat. It was four years ago. I had always lived a healthy lifestyle including a careful diet and regular exercise. I never smoked and had a yearly exam and Pap smear. But I began to have unusual abdominal pain and GI problems. My primary care doctor referred me to a gastroenterologist who referred me to a gynecologist and on and on it went! For over a year I was diagnosed and treated for everything from colitis to Crohn's disease to early menopause, but my symptoms only worsened. Finally, after countless tests, exploratory surgery was recommended. While waking up from the anesthetic I remember my surgeon telling me, "I am so very sorry, it is cancer and it is very advanced." My other memory is being wheeled past my husband Michael. He was leaning against the wall, sobbing. It was in this awful state that I was referred to Dr. Benigno.

"I have had chemotherapy and a recurrence requiring additional surgery including the removal of part of my colon.

Following this I had to have more chemotherapy. I am now cancer-free and a recent PET scan was negative.

"It is true that life looks very different after cancer. It's a struggle to find a new, changed version of yourself. I've walked with my husband hand in hand on our favorite beach again. We've celebrated holidays with our family and we've rescued more animals (my personal passion). And now I can stand before other cancer patients as living proof that one can beat it."

This patient now has several new passions: She constantly addresses women's groups and tells her story so that they understand the problems associated with the early diagnosis of ovarian cancer. She raises money for ovarian cancer research and frequently visits newly diagnosed patients who are just recovering from surgery. Her lovely and forceful presence takes away some of the fear and confusion and allows both hope and tranquility to devolve on such desperate situations. In all of these ventures she has earned my gratitude and respect.

DOROTHY

Patients can sometimes frighten oncologists for many reasons some of which are quite bizarre. I operated on a patient for ovarian cancer and in the postoperative period began what I thought would be a routine conversation. I told her that I recommended chemotherapy and as I began describing the drugs she interrupted me and told me that she would never consider taking chemotherapy. I was stunned by this response as she was young and healthy and had absolutely no contraindications to this treatment. When I asked her the reason for her refusal her answer was like a punch to the solar plexus. Her 19-year-old daughter had died of lymphoma the year before, and she told me that there was no way that she would ever consider taking chemotherapy as it would bring back memories that she would find unbearable.

A lengthy conversation ensued, during which she was completely in charge. I told her what any oncologist would have told her; your daughter's death is a very great tragedy but your death would neither cancel not expiate that tragedy. Other inane statements followed and each was met with the same intransigent refusal. She walked out of the office without a return appointment. I wrote her several letters reiterating my recommendation and informing her that I was worried about her ability to survive this illness without further treatment. I recommended that she see another oncologist for a second opinion. The letters went unanswered.

A year later her name appeared on the patient list for that morning and I entered the exam room slowly and with considerable trepidation. I expected to encounter someone who had been a beautiful and vibrant woman a year ago, transposed to a frail and wasted state. Not so! She looked better and younger and had not only a new job but also a new boyfriend. With a justifiably superior attitude she told me, "You see, I told you that I would make it." Not only was the physical examination normal, but so was the CT scan! She returns every year to tell me how wrong I was in my recommendations and next month will mark the *fifteenth* anniversary of the ignored advice!

This encounter has taught me that I do not have all the answers to the complicated puzzle surrounding one's ability to recover from a mortal illness. I had the slides from her surgery reviewed by another pathologist and there was no doubt at all; this was a Stage III cancer of the ovary. I can only surmise that this patient had a very powerful immune system that provided her with an exquisite self-induced treatment regimen. I hesitate to mention this as I have always maintained that when an oncologist talks about the immune response he or she has come to the end of understanding on a particular issue. Perhaps I need a keener insight into the complexity of the immune response.

Whether expressed or not, fear is an underlying emotion in all of these stories. Oncologists have a duty to try to help these patients to minimize this terror and one way to accomplish this is to divert attention away from the ministrations of the medical profession. Oncologists may make requests of patients that have nothing to do with medicine.

The first visit to my office is fraught with sheer terror and in an attempt to mollify that terror, I ask them to purchase next year's calendar—a large one with a different picture for every month and a big square enclosing each day. I ask them to circle the day corresponding to the first anniversary of our meeting and write in a plan to do something that they have always wanted to do. This produces two immediate effects:

First, it gives them something to look forward to that is a bit more pleasant than surgery and chemotherapy; second, it extends to them the subliminal message that I actually expect them to be around next year. A Men's Warehouse moment— *I guarantee it!* I also tell them that I am a very young doctor (unfortunately not true) and if you do well I look good. What is wrong with the physician giving the patient yet another reason to get well?

16

OUT-OF-THE-BOX TREATMENTS

What old people say you cannot do, you try and find that you can. Old deeds for old people, and new deeds for new.

—Henry David Thoreau

Do not follow where the path may lead. Go instead where there is no path and leave a trail.

—Ralph Waldo Emerson

WE ARE NOT doing as well as we ought to be doing. Advances in the treatment of ovarian cancer over the past quarter of a century have occurred incrementally: the addition of a step in the surgical procedure, a change in the dosage of a drug, or the addition of yet another drug to an already existing regimen. The results are not exactly met with a blast of trumpet music. In fact, I am so tired of reading journal articles that announce a several month improvement in progression-free survival in a small cohort of patients where the results are not statistically significant.

It is clear that a radical change will have to occur if we are to improve on the 70 percent to 80 percent recurrence rate. This will not happen until we enter the golden age of oncology where all cancers will be treated on the basis of individual changes in the nuclear protein peculiar to that patient's tumor. This would cause the instant death of all the cancer cells without harming a hair on the patient's head! Until this age is upon us we must make do with these out-of-the-box approaches, which hopefully will soon pass into the history of medicine under the heading of *barbaric treatments!*

1. **Cryo-ablation and Radiofrequency Ablation (RFA).** While a recurrent cancer of the ovary frequently involves widespread metastatic disease throughout the abdomen, it is sometimes localized to one area, which can be treated by an interventional radiologist. Metastatic lesions less than 4 or 5 centimeters located in the liver, kidney, adrenal gland, or lung are amenable to such treatment. A small needle is passed through the skin under CT guidance and goes through normal liver tissue and into the metastatic lesion. The RFA device, which consists of several wires attached to a current source, is then turned on. The heat produced causes apoptosis, or cell death, within the metastatic lesion. Cryo-ablation uses a similar approach, but with the use of gas to freeze the diseased tissue.

These treatments are referred to as percutaneous because the needle goes through the skin. This approach is the least invasive way of treating these lesions and allows for a fast recovery, limited hospital stay, and low cost. Unlike surgery, radiofrequency and cryo-ablation can be repeated easily if residual disease is present. Patients with two or more lesions in different lobes of the liver will not be candidates for surgery because of the amount of the liver that would have to be removed. Some studies suggest that RFA of a solitary liver metastasis less than 5 centimeters results in an excellent long-term survival.

Jason Levy, M.D., director of interventional radiology at Northside Hospital in Atlanta, has extensive experience in treating these metastatic lesions and is an industry innovator in establishing the use of radiofrequency and cryo-ablation in the treatment of ovarian cancer that has spread to these selected sites.

2. **Trans-Arterial Chemo-Embolization**. This technique involves the injection of chemotherapy directly into the hepatic artery, the artery that brings blood to the liver. This causes an ischemic effect which refers to a decrease in blood supply. This also causes a concentrated dose of chemotherapy to be placed directly into the metastatic lesion. When intra-arterial chemotherapy is performed, tumor drug concentrations constitute one or two orders of magnitude greater than what could be achieved by an intravenous infusion of chemotherapy. The dwell time of the drugs is markedly prolonged, and, because most of the drug is retained in the liver, systemic toxicity is

reduced. The reduction in blood supply produced by the occlusion of blood vessels works synergistically with the chemotherapy. It helps to overcome drug resistance by causing metabolically active cell membrane pumps to fail, thereby increasing intracellular retention of the chemotherapy drugs. This technique is also performed by the interventional radiologist.

3. **Selective Internal Radiation Therapy [SIRT].** This very new treatment for ovarian cancer metastatic to the liver involves the injection of a radioisotope called yttrium-90, which causes SIR microspheres to enter the liver lesion via the hepatic artery. The treatment is given on an outpatient basis with side effects much less than with conventional surgery. Because liver tumors tend to be very vascular, the infused microspheres become trapped in the small blood vessels which supply the tumor. Once trapped within the capillaries supplying the tumor, SIR microspheres irradiate the cancer cells and destroy the tumor while leaving the normal liver tissue relatively unscathed.

4. **Heated Intra-peritoneal Chemotherapy [HIPEC].** Primary as well as recurrent cancers of the ovary are usually confined to the abdominal cavity. The goal of surgery is to remove all of the cancer and when that occurs, there is a new option that involves the circulation of heated chemotherapy within the abdomen. Inflow and outflow tubes are placed in the abdomen and connected to a machine that is capable of heating and circulating the solution. The skin is temporarily closed with a suture and

the chemotherapy (usually Cisplatinum) mixed in two liters of saline is circulated at a temperature of around 43 degrees Celsius for ninety minutes. Following this the skin suture and tubes are removed and the abdominal cavity is copiously irrigated to remove all traces of the chemotherapy. The abdomen is then closed in the usual manner, thus completing the operation.

Although relatively new for ovarian cancer, HIPEC has been used for many years in the treatment of patients with colon and pancreatic cancer. It makes a great deal of sense to use this technique because cancer of the ovary is usually confined to the abdominal cavity when first diagnosed. However there is not yet enough data to support the routine use of HIPEC in patients with ovarian cancer.

5. **Trabectedin.** Penicillin came from the aspergillus mold and was discovered by Sir Alexander Fleming as a result of a laboratory error. Vincristine, a very powerful and widely used chemotherapy drug, came from the periwinkle plant. Trabectedin, derived from the lowly sea squirt which is a tubular sea animal, has been used in many medical studies. It binds to the DNA of the cancer cell and blocks the cell's ability to multiply, causing cell death and the shrinkage of tumors. This drug is approved in Europe for the treatment of soft tissue sarcomas and is now being tested in patients with ovarian cancer.

6. **Dendritic Vaccines.** For more than 100 years oncologists have dreamed of stimulating the immune response, thus

allowing the patient's body to become an instrument of treatment and healing. In the 1850s German physicians noticed that a patient's tumor would occasionally shrink if it became infected, leading to the concept that the body's own immune response could be used to fight cancer. Jenner's successful vaccine against small pox led to the belief that there could be a vaccine against cancer.

Toward the end of the 19th century, a pioneering New York surgeon named William Coley used a bacterial vaccine to treat inoperable sarcomas and achieved an astonishing 10 percent cure rate. He observed that producing fever was the key to tumor regression. In 1975 George Kohler and Cesar Milstein discovered how to make synthetic antibodies leading to the eventual discovery of *Herceptin,* an antibody-based drug widely used in the treatment of breast cancer.

A dendritic cell is an immune cell. There are several dendritic vaccine trials underway at the present time and I will briefly describe the one we are using in my practice. Mucins (high molecular weight proteins) have attracted attention as a potential target for immunotherapy because epithelial mucin surface antigen I (MUC I) is over-expressed in ovarian cancers up to forty times the level contained in normal cells. Remember, epithelial cells are found on the surface of the ovary and are the source of epithelial ovarian cancers.

Dendritic cell vaccination provides potent cells for the initiation of T-cell mediated immunity. The loading of dendritic cells with the MUC I fusion protein increases the specificity of the immune response. Specificity in this case refers to epithelial ovarian cancer specificity. T-cells are very powerful cells in the immune pathway. The dendritic cells are prepared from the patient's own white blood cells, which makes the process autologous (no foreign cells involved).

7. **Targeted Therapy.** All chemotherapy drugs are poisons and the dosage and interval between treatments are limited by the body's ability to tolerate the treatments. When the chemotherapy is given intravenously the same amount of the drug that reaches the skin of the elbow is what hits the tumor cells. It is as if there were several ants on the top of a precious piece of Meissen porcelain and one blasts the ants with a shotgun. The ants are destroyed but so is the porcelain. There is a considerable body of work devoted to methods of delivering drugs directly to the cancer cells while bypassing the normal cells, thus allowing massive doses of the drug to be introduced directly into the cancer without harming the patient. Numerous target and delivery systems are being tested and several clinical trials for targeted therapy are being conducted at various medical centers.

This review represents a discussion of only a few novel therapies available at the present time. As you might imagine, when there are so many treatment options there is not one that stands head and shoulders above the others and therefore it is necessary that the search for the "magic bullet" continues.

At the conclusion of a chapter that elucidates some out-of-the-box treatments, which may or may not fall into common usage at some future date, I am inspired to dwell for a moment on the accomplishments of one of history's legendary physicians. Moses Maimonides was born in Spain in 1135 and eventually settled in Egypt. He was a Rabbi before he studied medicine and he quickly became the most famous physician of his time. He wrote many treatises in medicine and philosophy and eventually became court physician to Saladin the Great. His intelligence and learning were so profound and his powers as a physician so unique that there exists, even to this day, the Jewish proverb, *From Moses to Moses there arose none like Moses*.

Saladin was the first Sultan of Egypt and Syria, and even after his prestigious appointment as the Sultan's personal physician, Maimonides continued working long hours treating patients from all walks of life and writing medical treatises that affected the practice of medicine for many centuries. I would give anything to gain an insight into one of his daily routines.

This little sojourn into the history of medicine teaches us that there is far more to the healing process than the vast number of treatments available to us at the present time. Maimonides could not take out an appendix, nor did he have access to penicillin, and yet his patients did very well. Perhaps his extraordinary capacity as a physician arose from his willingness to listen to his patients and transmit to them, through some subliminal process, his strong desire to see them get well. Maybe this is a common thread shared by the most effective physicians throughout the ages.

It is foolish for a modern physician to speculate on how a famous physician of another era would behave today. However, if Maimonides were practicing medicine now, I am certain of two things: First, he would be one of the leading physicians of our time; second, Moses Maimonides would never turn away a Medicare patient.

17

ALTERNATIVE MEASURES

IT IS PRECISELY because the literature on this subject is so vast that this chapter will be so brief. A trip to the medical section of a large bookstore will reveal numerous volumes dedicated to diet and nontraditional ways of treating many illnesses, including cancer. Browsing through the Internet provides us with a staggering list of remedies from aspirin to zinc. I cannot help but feel inadequate when I counsel patients to eat a healthy diet, avoid fast foods, and take vitamins. I recommend the services of a nutritionist—this gets me out of at least one of these difficulties.

It is believed that over 30 percent of patients with cancer seek some form of alternative treatment, either alone or in combination with standard therapy. Alternative medicine is an extremely broad and complex topic that is diverse in foundation as well as methodology. It ranges from diet and vitamin supplementation to mind-body alterations and Eastern practices devoted to concentration and relaxation. The term *integrative medicine* refers to a combination of conventional and alternative medicine and has become very popular in the United States. Andrew Weil is one of the leading exponents of integrative medicine and he stresses that it has the mission to restore the focus of medicine on health and healing while emphasizing the importance of the patient-physician relationship.

A patient with advanced cancer is captivated by an intrinsic terror that frequently leads to a search for "Something else out there." I lived and worked through the Laetrile era and I will describe this phenomenon in some detail as it will provide us with an insight into how desperate these patients can become. We all know that Laetrile is now discredited. I am by no means suggesting that this will be the fate of all alternative measures. I would, however, like to point out that these remedies do not undergo the rigorous scrutiny and testing that the FDA requires of chemotherapy drugs.

Laetrile is chemically related to amygdalin, a substance found naturally in the pits of apricots. Along with shark cartilage, this drug was extremely popular with cancer patients who sought nontraditional treatment. Laetrile was first isolated in 1830 by French chemists. In the presence of certain enzymes, amygdalin breaks down into a number of compounds including **cyanide!** It was first used as an anticancer drug in Germany in 1892, but was soon discontinued because it was too toxic. In the early 1950s Ernst Krebs began using a purified form of this drug in cancer patients. Although numerous animal and human studies have shown no benefit, the use of Laetrile continued well into the 1990s. We should always remember that patients obtained this drug at great expense.

Since there is no way for the consumer to be certain of the validity and usefulness of many forms of alternative medicine, there is a need for some sort of classification. Stephen Barrett, the founder and operator of Quackwatch, maintains that these health practices should be labeled as genuine, experimental, or questionable. I try not to lose sight of the fact that anything that a patient does under these circumstances may exert a placebo effect and therefore be of some value. When my patients discuss with me something that they would like to try along these lines, I investigate it as best I can, and, provided that it is not dangerous or does not interfere with ongoing treatment, I give it my benediction.

Edzard Ernst is a professor of complementary medicine and he and his colleagues have studied almost all forms of alternative medicine. He has concluded that most of these treatments, including acupuncture, herbal medicine, homeopathy, and reflexology, are statistically indistinguishable from placebo treatments. No fewer than four Nobel Laureates have criticized the lack of proper scientific investigation that accompanied the support given to alternative medicine by the National Institutes of Health!

I find it difficult to criticize many nontraditional forms of treatment mainly because of my knowledge of the development of penicillin. As pointed out earlier, it was derived from the common aspergillus mold, something that was probably rubbed on infected areas of the body for centuries, producing excellent results. I wonder how many people in the traditional medical community in those days disapproved of the earliest use of penicillin because it was not *standard of care.*

I refer my patients to a community support group associated with my hospital. In addition to counseling them about diet, herbs, and other nontraditional approaches to healing, this excellent and very professional organization provides the following services:

- Wellness Workout
- Yoga
- T'ai Chi
- Pilates
- Zumba
- Music Therapy
- Meditation
- Art Therapy

It is hard to believe that there is a patient with cancer who would not benefit greatly from many of these services. In an effort to "cover all the bases," I see to it that my patients are referred to this support group. Not only do they receive wonderful help in many different disciplines, but the sessions are open and confer the added benefit of group therapy.

Patients seek alternative remedies not only to improve their chances for survival but also to run away from traditional treatments that can be overwhelming and frightening. A patient with an advanced cancer may have an unreasonable expectation for the ability of current treatment modalities to produce a favorable outcome. Bernard Lown, a Nobel Prize–winning physician, wrote an extraordinary book titled *The Lost Art of Healing*. It contains a sentence that startled me in its simplicity and relevance. "The childish faith in the magic of technology is one reason the American public has tolerated inhumane doctoring." This is a tragic indictment of the medical profession by one its most revered members, and, as such, it serves as a constant reminder that oncologists must try to balance the potential benefits of a treatment regimen with the severity of its side effects.

18

THE HUSBAND FACTOR

LET ME BEGIN by telling you that I have found most husbands to be extremely helpful in the care of my patients. While I pointed out instances when I was asked if the cancer was contagious and had to endure a recitation of the spouse's own symptoms, these encounters are unusual and were mentioned to point out the downside side of the spectrum. There is one encounter, however, that I will never forget and I will share it with you with considerable and justifiable reticence. As mentioned before, it is sometimes necessary to take out part of the colon so that the cancer is removed in its entirety. Many years ago, because of the extent of the tumor, I had to remove half of the colon. When I finished the operation and relayed this information to her husband, his remark startled me. "So I guess this means that I'm now married to a semicolon!" I don't have a night job writing dark humor for television shows. This is a direct quotation.

My wife once told me that she married me for better or for worse but not for lunch, unless, of course, the lunch was in a restaurant. I had some misgivings about writing this chapter, but since the husband is such an important part of the caregiving equation, I decided to proceed. As a young physician I soon learned that I needed to relate to the spouse, and that husband and wife did not always see things through the same optic. Husbands are frequently more confused and frightened than the patients themselves and I have found that it can take considerable effort to reach out to them so that they can actually become as helpful as they want to be.

By far the most difficult husbands that I encounter are the engineers. For an engineer, there is always an answer. No sane person would ever contemplate building a bridge from San Francisco to Tokyo, but an engineer would attempt to explain how it could be possible. They ask me how their wives are going to do after chemotherapy and when I tell them that I don't know, they sometimes tell me that they want another opinion!

Primum non nocere (first do no harm) is medicine's first and greatest admonition, and all physicians learn this in their first year of medical school. *Be thou not judgmental* is another important admonition, only this one was not taught in school and I had to learn it the hard way. When I encounter pitched battles in my office I have to remind myself that I am not a marriage counselor. At the heart of many of these conflicts lies the issue of control. No matter how one spins it, another person has entered the relationship and in my case it is a man.

This is unusual, but there are times when this is more of a problem than it ought to be.

I return phone calls in the following manner when it is the husband who answers the phone: "Hello, this is Benedict Benigno, may I please speak with your wife?" I cannot tell you the level of angst that envelops me when the husband begins to recite his wife's symptoms, including, on occasion, minute details of the menstrual cycle! This, of course, is quite unusual, and I find that it tests both comprehension and tolerance. Lord Chesterfield, in one of his famous letters to his son, wrote that a gentleman is never rude except on purpose. With that in mind, I interrupt and ask to speak directly with my patient!

Marriages have literally disintegrated in front of me, and it is these episodes that have inspired the writing of this chapter. On a number of occasions husbands have left their wives in the middle of chemotherapy, sometimes with the rather flippant remark, "I'm out of here." Surgery and the administration of chemotherapy are far easier for me than an attempt to keep so fragile a patient from dissolving and simply giving up. It represents the supreme moment of vulnerability and raises loneliness to an unspeakable level. I cannot imagine what it must be like after a chemotherapy session to return to a home devoid of the person with whom one has been living for twenty years. Simon and Garfunkel had a song in the '60s that contained the words, "Silence like a cancer grows." I can find no other way to put it—this is a double dose of cancer!

All marriages acquire varying degrees of stress over the years and a chronic and mortal illness increases the stress by a quantum leap. If someone is diagnosed with a pancreatic cancer that has spread to the liver and lung, almost without exception death will ensue in a matter of months. The spouse hardly has time to adjust to the diagnosis before it is over. Stress in such cases derives from illness and impending death and has its own inherent time frame. A recurrent cancer of the ovary is another matter entirely. Numerous rounds of repetitive chemotherapy are sometimes punctuated by surgical procedures, all of which bring some patients and their marriages to the breaking point. Even the best of relationships can crumble in the wake of such disaster.

Cancer! The removal of ones sexual organs! Castration! Infertile! Menopausal! Chemotherapy! Bald! Vomiting! Anemic! And then the sucker leaves! Only recently I heard the poignant words, "Dr. Benigno, I have nothing to look forward to. Who is going to sign up for this?" The most gratifying moments in my career have occurred when I have seen women return from this very dark place, become healthy again and find relationships more meaningful than their previous marriages. In this, as in many other things, the secret is to turn adversity into triumph.

19

THE BIOLOGIC AND GENETIC BACKGROUND OF OVARIAN CANCER

Human beings are ultimately nothing but carriers—passageways—for genes. They ride us into the ground like racehorses from generation to generation. Genes don't think about what constitutes good or evil. They don't care whether we are happy of unhappy. We're just means to an end for them. They only think about what is most efficient for them.

—*1Q84*
Haruki Murakami
Japanese writer and translator

DNA IS THE very foundation of a cell. In the overall scheme of things, a person is totally irrelevant to the process of life except as a participant in the transmission of DNA from one generation to the next. We are personal and DNA is not.

DNA is interested in DNA. Once we produce children and raise them to the point where they can become parents themselves, we are then totally irrelevant to life's grand scheme. It is the DNA and not the person that is guilty of supreme egotism. This is where science enters the domain of philosophy and assigns to mankind the status of carrier pigeon! In the world of cells, the cancer cell has become king of the mountain because it alone is immortal. It is so depressing that the only living thing that has the audacity to capture immortality is the cancer cell.

A single cell is a very exciting structure. It carries within it the capacity to divide into another normal cell or to begin the process whereby it is transformed into a cancer cell. All cells have the capacity for malignant transformation and the intense study that revolves around this process is the very foundation of present day cancer research. The mechanism whereby normal cells stop dividing into other normal cells and begin their journey into cancer cells is an extremely complicated process. Many disparate scientific branches are trying to solve this problem and in so doing, capture oncology's grandest prize.

Some of these issues are easy to understand; for instance, the relationship of cigarette smoking to cancer of the lung and the relationship of the sexually transmitted HPV virus to cancer of the cervix. People who work in aniline dye factories have a high incidence of bladder cancer. But the etiology of most cancers, such as ovarian cancer, remains ill-understood.

The cancer process is related to the aging process in that the older we become the more likely we are to get a cancer. All men who live long enough will get prostate cancer.

The following outline will give the reader a brief insight into some of the precipitating factors in the development of a cancer cell.

TUMOR SUPPRESSOR GENES

In a perfect world all cells would contain genes that would suppress the ability of a cell to undergo malignant transformation. None of these genes would ever undergo a deleterious mutation and no one would ever get cancer. Many complex mechanisms prevent a normal cell from mutating into a cancer cell and chief among these are the tumor suppressor genes, a group of genes that "puts the brakes" on cancer development.

When DNA damage is detected in a cell some tumor suppressor genes can stop the cell from dividing until the damage is repaired. When these genes function perfectly, cells with damaged DNA are made to commit "cell suicide" or apoptosis. When tumor suppressor genes undergo a deleterious mutation and do not function properly, the cells with DNA damage continue to divide with subsequent daughter cells retaining the same DNA damage until a cancerous tumor emerges. The cell cycle is the mechanism whereby the old cells in an organ are replaced by identical normal cells. When the DNA code of a tumor suppressor gene is altered, there is no longer a tumor suppressor signal that is recognized by the cell. It is this mal-communication on a cellular level that begins the process leading to the development of a cancer cell.

BRCA 1 AND BRCA 2

BRCA 1 and BRCA 2 are by far the most important tumor suppressor genes with respect to breast and ovarian cancers. As mentioned, BRCA is an acronym for breast cancer. Deleterious mutations on the BRCA 1 and BRCA 2 genes are found in 10 percent to 15 percent of all epithelial ovarian cancers. The lifetime risk of developing an ovarian cancer in mutation carriers is up to 40 percent in the BRCA 1 gene mutation group and 10 percent to15 percent in the BRCA 2 gene mutation group. Women who are of Ashkanazi descent and have a deleterious mutation on BRCA 1 will have a 70 percent lifetime risk of developing ovarian cancer! BRCA-related familial ovarian cancers have genetically distinct clones involving many locations. These cancers progress faster but are more sensitive to platinum-based chemotherapy and are also more likely to respond to PARP inhibitors.

As in familial breast cancers, an inactivated allele (alternative form of a gene) is inherited by the cells, and the loss of BRCA 1 or BRCA 2 function occurs in the ovarian cancer cells through the loss of heterozygosity of the normal allele. Heterozygosity occurs when there are different alleles on a specific chromosomal site. Cells that lose the BRCA genes repair DNA by error-producing mechanisms, leading to chromosomal rearrangements and genetic instability. Ovarian cancer cells with mutations of BRCA 1 and BRCA 2 are less able to repair damaged DNA caused by platinum chemotherapy. A major cause of resistance to platinum chemotherapy may arise from these mutations.

A woman's lifetime risk of developing breast cancer is 12 percent (120 out of 1,000) but the incidence increases to 60 percent (600 out of 1,000) in those patients with a harmful BRCA mutation. The lifetime risk of developing ovarian cancer is 1.4 percent (14 out of 1,000), which increases to 15 percent to 40 percent (150 to 400 out of 1,000) with the BRCA mutation. Mutations occur in many other genes, but the mutations in the BRCA genes are by far the most important.

ONCOGENES

Oncogenes are genes that have the ability to cause a cancer to develop. The first oncogene was discovered in 1970 by Dr. G. Steve Martin at the University of California, Berkeley. It was found in a chicken retrovirus and was called *src* (pronounced *sarc* as in *sarcoma*). A retrovirus is a virus whose genes are encoded in RNA instead of DNA. In 1976 Drs. J. Michael Bishop and Harold E. Varmus demonstrated that oncogenes were defective proto-oncogenes. These are normal genes that can become oncogenes due to mutation. They are found in many organisms, including humans. For this extraordinary work they were awarded the Nobel Prize in physiology in 1989. The best review of oncogenes and cancer that I have encountered to date was written by Dr. Carlo M. Croce [N

Engl J Med 2008; 358:502-511] and will be widely quoted in this section.

More than fifteen oncogenes have been identified in ovarian cancers. Most normal cells undergo a programmed form of death called apoptosis. Activated oncogenes can interdict this process and cause those cells that ought to die to survive and proliferate. Most oncogenes require an additional step, such as a mutation in another gene, or an environmental factor, such as a viral infection, in order to cause the development of a cancer. Oncogenes are activated by chromosomal rearrangement, mutation, and gene amplification. Many cancer drugs target the proteins encoded by these oncogenes. A proto-oncogene can become an oncogene by a relatively small modification of its original function. Oncogenes encode proteins that control cell proliferation, apoptosis, or both.

What is so frightening about all of this is that inherent in every one of our cells is the potential for a mutation into a cancer cell as a result of the transformation of a proto-oncogene into an oncogene. All cancers are caused by alterations in oncogenes, tumor suppressor genes, or microRNA genes. A single genetic change is rarely responsible for the development of a malignant tumor. Multiple steps including sequential alterations in several oncogenes must occur before the appearance of a clinically detectable cancer.

Let us use the architectural plans of a building as a metaphor for understanding the difference between DNA and RNA. DNA is the master plan for the entire structure. RNA refers to component parts such as the electrical plans, the plumbing plans, etc. DNA is identical in all of the body's cells; RNA is as different in liver cells and pancreas cells as it is different in kidney cells and colon cells, etc. MicroRNA is a small RNA molecule that may function as an oncogene OR a tumor suppressor gene depending on its environment. This means that it has the capacity to augment or suppress the development of a cancer cell. MicroRNA may be very important in the transportation of cancer-killing treatments directly into the cancer cell. This is the very essence of targeted therapy and is one of the most exciting cancer treatments on the horizon.

In addition to the initial clones and sub-clones, tumors can also contain progenitor or stem cells. These cells can differ in sensitivity to chemotherapy and actually contribute to the high rate of recurrence in ovarian cancer. Stem cells comprise less than 1 percent of the population of ovarian cancer cells and are extremely resistant to standard chemotherapy. The development of drugs that would specifically target these stem cells would represent a major advance in the management of patients with ovarian cancer. For these reasons, the initiating steps in the development of a cancer on the genetic and molecular level are of great clinical importance as we struggle for more efficacious and less toxic forms of treatment.

No oncologist is an island. The next generation of treatments will emerge from the basic science laboratory and, indeed, in the near future, the treating physician may very well be replaced by the molecular biologist! Oncogenes are of vital importance in the ongoing efforts to develop targeted therapy, which will be an interim treatment prior to that glorious moment when the basic scientist becomes *Maestro* and ascends, baton in hand, to oncology's podium!

Leukemia gives us an insight into the role of oncogenes in cancer initiation and progression. When chronic myelogenous leukemia converts to acute leukemia, the malignant clone acquires an additional t(9;22) translocation, an isochromosome 17 or trisomy of chromosome 8. When follicular lymphoma becomes aggressive, the lymphoma cells often bear a t(8;14) translocation in addition to the original t(14;18) translocation. These findings support the theory that most hematopoietic (blood) cancers are initiated by the activation of an oncogene followed by alterations in tumor suppressor genes. I have tried very hard, but there is no way I could simplify the above information.

In contrast, most cancers, including epithelial ovarian cancers, are initiated by a loss of function of a tumor suppressor gene followed by alterations in oncogenes. This represents a polar opposite of the initiating factors in hematopoietic cancers such as leukemia. These basic differences on a genetic level are of pristine importance as newer ways of treating cancer, especially in the arena or personalized medicine, are being developed in laboratories around the world.

Everyone knows that the *War on Cancer* evolved during the Nixon administration and that it has cost hundreds of billions of dollars to date. What most people do not know is the ferocity of the belligerent behind-the-scenes arguments that occurred while the battle plan for this war was being drawn up. The medical profession felt that the best way to conquer cancer was to devise more radical surgical procedures, build bigger radiation therapy machines, and develop more potent chemotherapy regimens, all of which would take patients to the very limit of the body's endurance.

James Watson, the co-discoverer of the double helix structure of DNA, was a strident and vociferous member of the scientific community who argued for the war to be waged in the molecular and genetics laboratories. Watson received the Nobel Prize in Medicine in 1962. Even with such a strong and famous exponent of the basic science contingent, they wound up losing to the clinicians. The era of bigger and more toxic oncology had begun. I personally believe that if Watson's group had won, we would now be working in the golden age of oncology. The ultra-radical surgical procedures and the extreme toxicity of the newer forms of chemotherapy would be relegated to the historic perspective of the *Barber Surgeons*.

Does the reader know the origin or that term? In the Middle Ages, surgery was performed by the barbers! After each operation they would wrap the bloody bandages around white poles in front of their shops to dry them so that the dirty and infected bandages could be used for the next customer! To this day, the international symbol of the barber shop is a wide, red diagonal stripe running down a white pole. I think that I would prefer a shampoo and a little off the top!

20

A POSTPARTUM TRAGEDY

Out, damn'd spot! Out, I say! Yet who would have thought the old man to have had so much blood in him?

—William Shakespeare, *Macbeth*
Lady Macbeth's Soliloquy

That heaven should practice stratagems upon so soft a subject as myself?

—William Shakespeare, *Romeo and Juliet*
Juliet's Lament

NANCY'S STORY

LADY MACBETH SPEAKS these famous words after she has killed the king. All patients with ovarian cancer share the same sentiment, wanting the tumor out yesterday. I frequently mumble in the operating room, "Who would have thought this patient to have had so much cancer in her?" No one has ever pronounced life fair, but the gradations that occur along the road can be startling. We are supposed to die before our children but not when they are in pre-kindergarten. Such a tragedy throws life's time clock out of sync and visits upon the mother her most primal fears. All cancers that are associated with pregnancy are worse and carry a poorer prognosis precisely because of the pregnancy. The vastly increased blood supply to most organs augurs a greater chance of blood-borne metastases.

There are certain conditions that should represent an oncologic "no-fly" zone and at the top of this list are cancers that affect children and pregnant woman. Ovarian cancer is quite rare in pregnancy and I have encountered it only four times in my long career. It produces changes in the woman's psyche that transcend fear and concern over one's own mortality. The constant thought of not seeing your own children grow up produces an ineffable sadness and pathos worthy of a Greek tragedy.

Nancy was not only pregnant, but, unbeknownst to everyone including her doctors, she also had an advanced cancer of the ovary. The caesarean section produced a beautiful baby boy and both mother and child left the hospital two days later after an uncomplicated postoperative course. The family, united again, settled into an ageless routine of feedings, diapers, and visits to the pediatrician. This was her second child and there was nothing unusual in the beginning. Her strength returned quickly and she was enjoying her new baby immensely

What was about to happen was as far removed from her thoughts as a walk on the moon. Several months after the delivery she began to notice that the scar from her recent C-section was getting larger instead of disappearing as expected. This was ascribed to inflammation and when the prescribed treatment not only did not work, but was also accompanied by additional swelling and discomfort, she insisted on a CT scan. The report was devastating in the extreme—a large mass in the ovary with widespread metastatic disease, including a number of nodular masses in the upper abdomen near the liver and spleen.

People in their 80s become disjointed by such news. This woman was in her early 30s and, because she was the mother of two small children, she became more terrified by the thought of not being around for them than about her diagnosis and impending treatment. In one of Rainer Maria Rilke's poems he asks the question, "Who is pulling at the strings of my heart–how sweet is the song?" Cancer does not pull at the strings; it yanks at them and the song is a dirge!

She was referred to me after three cycles of chemotherapy with Carboplatinum and Taxol, which were given intravenously. I performed an extensive operation that removed not only the uterus, tubes, and ovaries but also the omentum and the lower abdominal wall where the tumor had invaded the scar from the caesarian section. She recovered well from the extensive surgery and went on to finish the chemotherapy regimen. I never get a warm fuzzy feeling about how someone with such an advanced cancer of the ovary is going to do. Unfortunately, in her case the outcome was neither warm nor fuzzy as she developed the worst of all possible recurrences.

Because of a severe headache, she went to the emergency room where a CT scan showed brain metastases. She received radiation treatments to the entire brain and because of a lingering tumor in the region of the cerebellum she was treated with stereotactic radiation, which is a method of delivering radiation in high doses to specific areas.

The treatment was successful and follow-up scans of the brain over two years later remained negative. The disease eventually spread to the spleen, requiring a splenectomy and additional chemotherapy. Repeat imaging studies showed extensive liver metastases, requiring yet another change in chemotherapy. Shortly after the last change in chemotherapy, she finally stopped working, much of the sparkle went out of her eyes, and she went home from the hospital and died in the loving arms of a family benumbed by the tragic and bitter briefness of her days.

21

JESSICA AND THE WILL TO LIVE— A BELATED EPITAPH FOR A GREAT LADY

> *Here, darling, take these rags*
> *That once were tender flesh.*
> *I tore it up, I wore it down–*
> *All I have now are these two wings.*
>
> —Marina Tsvetayeva
> Twentieth-Century Russian Poet

CANCER SURGEONS DO not always have the luxury of preparing their patients for surgery. Indeed, we sometimes meet them for the first time when they are on the operating room table fully anesthetized with the abdomen already opened. Such was my encounter with Jessica, whose surgery began with the presumptive diagnosis of a benign fibroid tumor of the uterus, which proved to be an advanced cancer of the ovary. I was called to the operating room and completed the operation and removed all of the cancer without the formality of an informed consent. I went ahead under the assumption that she would have given me the green light.

The next morning I entered her room and introduced myself. "I'm Benedict Benigno and I operated on you yesterday. They found a cancer of the ovary and because I am a gynecologic oncologist, your doctor asked me to come to the operating room and complete the procedure. I was able to remove all the cancer but it will be necessary for you to have chemotherapy. I would be happy to ask one of my patients, who sat where you are sitting ten years ago, to visit you and share her experiences with you. I will also help you to get another opinion if this is something that would make things easier for you at this time."

I have not found a better way to talk to people in such circumstances. All information is imparted in short, clear sentences at the end of which is an infusion of hope in the person of a patient who long ago had a similar problem and who would be willing to introduce herself and act as educator and cheerleader. Former patients communicate in a different manner than oncologists and there is no more powerful message than the introduction of someone who has beaten back the beast many years ago.

The diagnosis of cancer benumbs both patient and oncologist alike, but of course in extremely different ways. Physicians must find a way to help these patients become anterior to their illness which is the first step on the road to placing it in a proper bucket and putting a lid on it. I now find that most of my patients are younger than I am leading me to toy with the idea that maybe the ancient Greeks were right—there are gods on Mount Olympus and we are their theater. If it is all theater then let us try to move from tragedy to comedy.

As mentioned earlier, a sense of humor in a physician can be very therapeutic, but, unfortunately, there is little room for it during the first encounter. Jessica kept staring at me during the conversation and I could not help noticing that her eyes appeared to be getting larger, the only sign of emotion that I could detect. When I finished speaking she looked at me, and in a very calm voice devoid of either sorrow or anger, she simply told me that she was going to live for another six years. When I asked her why she chose six years, she told me that she was divorced, her husband was untraceable and her only child was a junior in high school and he would graduate college in six years.

This conversation occurred many years before I was able to understand that a patient's psyche and the very complicated mental mechanisms that constitute will and the processing of issues relevant to survival have a great deal to do with someone's ability to triumph over a very serious illness. These concepts are nebulous at best, and are extremely difficult to study. I no longer believe that personality type devolves on either the development of cancer or its outcome. However, it is intriguing that such things as fear, anger, and even the ability to ignore the problem entirely, might have an effect, one way or the other, on the body's ability to modify the effects of a cancer. To this day oncologists do not understand cancer's compass; disease and treatment are aligned but outcome is multidirectional.

Jessica was treated with chemotherapy and four years later developed a recurrence that required additional surgery and chemotherapy. Another recurrence responded equally well to yet another treatment regimen. Several months after her son graduated from college she died. This story is a very good example of how patients can play a major role in their recovery and longevity, and that physicians should never presume that a good outcome is entirely due to their efforts.

22

A LONG OVERDUE CHANGE

Full fathom five thy father lies;
Of his bones are coral made;
Those are pearls that were his eyes:
Nothing of him that doth fade,
But doth suffer a sea-change
Into something rich and strange.

—William Shakespeare, *The Tempest*
Ariel's Song

SLASH, BURN, AND poison are oncology's ignoble triad—slash being surgery, burn being radiation therapy, and, of course, poison refers to chemotherapy. We are approaching the 70th anniversary of the advent of chemotherapy, and surgery and radiation therapy have been with us for well over 100 years. This conjures up the primal scream of my New York childhood— **"Enough already!"**

I can think of no better destiny for oncology than a sea change into something rich and strange. Smallpox was mankind's scourge until Edward Jenner vaccinated the Empress

Catherine against this disease, giving the process great credibility. Polio terrified parents and almost destroyed the career of Franklin Roosevelt and now, thanks to the Salk vaccine, this is a disease of historical interest only. All of the newer forms of therapy described in previous chapters are merely interim dalliances, things to think about until **IT** comes along. Just exactly what this "it" is no one seems to know.

Cellular biologists talk about translational research and the manner in which cells talk to one another and turn each other on or off. Geneticists describe the molecular structure of cancer and how cancer behaves on a molecular level. Soon, the specific organ of origin will no longer be important, as all cancers will be treated according to their individual molecular profile. Certain cancers of the pancreas will be treated in the same manner in which certain cancers of the ovary are treated. The quest for such a personalized method of treatment is at the heart of all of the exciting basic science research which, hopefully, will soon bring us into a therapeutic renaissance.

All cancers are currently treated based on where they originate. Gynecologic oncologists operate on patients with ovarian cancer, colorectal surgeons operate on patients with colon cancer, etc. Chemotherapy regimens are constructed along strict guidelines with respect to the organ from which the cancer arose. What is now known on a cellular and molecular level makes me believe that such approaches are rather inane and are on the way out. I will now make an attempt to guide the reader toward what is coming down the road.

Present-day chemotherapy is "shotgun medicine" for two very important reasons: The drugs go in equal doses to both cancer cells and normal cells; all patients will receive the same regimen based on the patient's cancer diagnosis and stage. In the first instance all patients are underserved. In the latter instance we know that a certain percentage of patients are doomed to fail the most popular treatment and yet it is not possible to predict which patients will fall into this category. We also know that certain drugs showed spectacular success in a small number of patients with a particular cancer, and yet these drugs were never approved because of their poor performance in the majority of cases. The potential of these "poor performers" to produce a successful result in those patients who fail standard therapy is unknown.

For many years, attempts have been made to choose chemotherapy drugs based on chemo-sensitivity testing done on tumor tissue removed at the time of surgery. Such testing is not yet as accurate as we would like it to be and has not passed into the mainstream. New molecular testing methods are emerging, which include testing for specific genes, proteins, and somatic mutations in cancer cells. Hopefully, these testing methods will allow the oncologist to better define prognosis on a more scientific level and to recommend treatment options that are more likely to succeed for an individual patient.

Molecular information derived from the patient's tissue will be entered into a database, which will include past history, family history, physical findings, and imaging studies. This will contribute to decisions related to treatment and prognosis. In the future all cancers will be classified on a molecular basis and this classification will be completely independent of the organ which contains the cancer. For the past 150 years such classifications were made by pathologists who look at the microscopic slides of the cancers through a light microscope. Oncology is not the only specialty that will undergo radical transformation.

Translational research is a new field embracing genomics, proteomics, and metabolomics, and looks at the contributions of genes, proteins, and metabolic pathways to human physiology. It is a variation in these pathways that can lead to serious illness. This is a good example of how modern science requires a team approach and not just the efforts of a single scientist working in a narrow field. These disciplines require a vast knowledge in bioinformatics, molecular modeling, and simulation. Research in personalized medicine will identify individual solutions based on the susceptibility profile of the individual patient.

We can all feel, if not actually hear, the hoof beats of radical change approaching. Although in its infancy, targeted therapy is beginning to take shape. Herceptin is now used in the treatment of women with breast cancer in which the protein HER2 is over-expressed. Gleevec is a drug that inhibits the enzyme tyrosine kinase and is used to treat those chronic myeloid leukemias that have the BCR-ABL fusion gene, which is the product of a reciprocal translocation between chromosome 9 and chromosome 22. As you might imagine these concepts are as difficult as they are exciting and they represent a radical departure from traditional medicine. I apologize for the scientific pyrotechnics. I was not able to simplify this paragraph!

23

A TOLSTOY MOMENT

I go, and it is done; the bell invites me.
Hear it not, Duncan, for it is a knell
That summons thee to heaven or to hell.

—William Shakespeare, *Macbeth*
Act II

NOTHING THAT I have ever read has more precisely crystallized what it is like to get a cancer and then to die from it, than Tolstoy's short story, *The Death of Ivan Ilyich*. It is all there— the totally normal and boring life that precedes the vague initial symptoms, the full-blown terror as the pain worsens, the insouciance of the physicians, the startling changes in family dynamics, and then the loneliness, pain, and horror surrounding death. Tolstoy portrays the protagonist as a dreary social-climbing bureaucrat unhappily married with children. His comfortable existence is punctuated by moves to several locations to further his career, and his self-assured life is devoid of either passion or meaning. In the words of Henry David Thoreau, he is leading a life of quiet desperation.

And then it happens, starting as a vague pain in the abdomen, which is intermittent and dismissed as something minor and fleeting. However, the pain returns with a vengeance, and concern quickly transcends into sheer terror prompting, at his wife's insistence, a visit to a "famous doctor." We get a marvelous glimpse into medicine as it was practiced toward the end of the 19th century with endless poking, auscultation, and thumping followed by a bizarre discussion in the consulting room. "It is either the appendix or a floating kidney!" I did not know that they could float! The patient only wants to know if it is serious and he never gets an answer to this simple and very important question. The pain worsens and then becomes unbearable, requiring the frequent administration of narcotics.

At first Ivan Ilyich is able to continue working as a judge, coming into court everyday, but soon his colleagues notice what he has been desperately trying to keep hidden, and it is apparent to him that he is unable to keep working. His coworkers patronize him and can scarcely conceal their wish that he retire. This part of the story teaches us how much work serves to identify who we are, and how important it is for patients to continue working during their treatments.

In a startling sentence the author talks about the sensation of being a passenger on a train that begins to move, producing the inability to tell whether the train is moving forward or backward. This is a fundamental question peculiar to all patients with a life-threatening illness; am I getting better or am I regressing? Ivan Ilyich saw several physicians and never got any direct answers. All he wanted was some simple information. What is happening to me? Am I going to get better or am I going to die? What treatment do you recommend? The progression of his disease is recounted brilliantly as the extraordinary degree of his pain induces him to have a servant hold his legs up in the air as he tries all kinds of remedies when the ministrations of the medical profession fail to help him. He can no longer find comfort in his bed and starts to live on the sofa.

Prior to his illness it is apparent that his relationship with his wife has become tepid at best. However, as the disease progresses dislike becomes transformed into a hatred that knows no bounds. His wife asks the simple question, "Are you better tonight," and this produces in him an unspeakable rage followed by a not very polite dismissal. His daughter, recently engaged to the man of her dreams, has no patience for her father's behavior and tells her mother that she pities her father but does not see how they are responsible for what is happening to him. The father senses this and completely understands that he is ruining their lives. In addition to the issues of pain and impending death, he must now deal with the guilt associated with the devastation that the illness is bringing to his family.

He finally dies but not before three full days of howling in the throes of a level of pain that has no name. It is very interesting that toward the end it is pain, and not the fear of death, that is the all-consuming issue. It appears that fear is in inverse proportion to the square of the distance from death. This short story provides such a brilliant insight into family dynamics in the home of a dying person. I believe that any oncologist could have written it!

I have to realize that when my patients come to the office I may not always have an accurate perception of the family problems that the illness has produced. Relationships are complicated enough without the unimaginable difficulties produced by a terminal illness. Since ovarian cancer may drag on for many years, even the best of marriages can be transported to the edge. Family issues are not always brought to the attention of the oncologist. Perhaps questions pertinent to these problems should be part of the record of each office visit.

Susan Sontag has written that it is not death that we fear, but degradation. She lived in the shadow of cancer for most of her adult life and her views on cancer and death are brilliantly recounted in her wonderful book *Illness as Metaphor*. We all accept death intellectually. It is its imminence that induces terror.

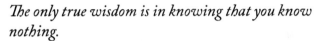

24

IS IT REALLY TRUE?

> *The only true wisdom is in knowing that you know nothing.*
>
> —Socrates

> *Logic will get you from A to B. Imagination will take you everywhere.*
>
> —Albert Einstein

TRUTH, I AM told, is anything that continues. The telephone call from John McDonald came on a Friday afternoon and began with a request for a Z-Pack because he was feeling under the weather. He asked that the prescription be called in to the pharmacy under his wife's name because he did not want it on his record that his physician was a gynecologist! I told him that this was illegal and that I would have to give his name to the pharmacist but that it would be highly unlikely that such sordid information would make the front page of the local newspaper. He accepted this explanation with some reticence and then, almost as an aside, he told me that he had some very good news.

It seemed that the final analysis of the data showed that our test picked up all of the stage one ovarian cancers. He went on to say that I was not to tell anyone until the article indicating the phenomenal accuracy of our test for ovarian cancer was published. I immediately informed him of the Sicilian code of *omerta*, which in effect means silence until death! I was unable to contain the exuberance that enveloped me and yet he relayed this momentous news as though he were describing a trip to the supermarket. Have two more dissimilar people ever collaborated on a research project?

I had a great deal of difficulty processing this information. The very morning of the phone call I saw three new patients in the office who had advanced cancer of the ovary who would require an unimaginable amount of surgery and chemotherapy. All of them had Stage III disease and were leading perfectly normal lives until a week or two prior to their CT scans. Would this mean that all women at the time of their annual physical examination and Pap smear could have an ovarian cancer screening test done on a single drop of blood which could be positive in Stage I disease, or perhaps before the actual transition into a cancer? May all your dreams come true is an ancient Chinese curse!

Making some impact on the immense devastation of ovarian cancer was the greatest of my dreams when I began my career many years ago and, now that it was possibly at hand, I was transported to another realm. If the Chinese are right then this is a curse that I would gladly endure! I imagined the end of the surgery that I was so assiduously trained to perform and I envisioned the chemotherapy shelves gathering dust. However, I am experienced enough to realize that it might become quite a battle to bring this test into the reality of current practice without the laborious efforts of phase one testing, repetitive publication, and the byzantine pathways leading to FDA approval.

This great good news gave me cause to reflect on the history of the Ovarian Cancer Institute and the future directions that, with a little bit of luck, might enable us to make contributions to the knowledge not only of ovarian cancer but to the process of cancer itself. Who is to say that major breakthroughs must come from famous research centers? As of the writing of this chapter, John McDonald is working on a panel of drugs that can kill the progenitor or stem cells, which are notoriously resistant to chemotherapy and which are responsible for the unacceptably high recurrence rate in ovarian cancer. All cancers have progenitor cells and that is why this work is so exciting.

25

FREQUENTLY ASKED QUESTIONS

*A woman's life is like a great house full of rooms...
and in the innermost room, the holy of holies, the
soul sits alone and waits for a footstep that never
comes.*

Edith Wharton, *"The Fullness of Life"*

Why does a woman get cancer of the ovary?

There is no good answer to this question. Unlike the relationship of cigarette smoking to cancer of the lung, there is not a specific carcinogen related to this disease. Having one's first child after the age of 35, obesity, and a positive family history as well as deleterious mutations on the BRCA 1 and BRCA 2 genes are important factors. However, most women in this category will *not* get ovarian cancer. Taking the birth control pill for over five years will confer an enormous protection against this cancer. Lifestyle plays little if any role in the etiology of this cancer. A routine annual visit to the gynecologist is of limited value in this illness and the Pap smear is totally useless. A positive Pap smear has led me to the diagnosis of ovarian cancer only three times in my career. Please remember that in 10,000 annual visits to a gynecologist, an ovarian cancer will be diagnosed but one time! There is no way to screen for ovarian cancer until a new diagnostic test comes along that is 100 percent accurate.

If you have symptoms of bloating and cramping abdominal pain, especially after eating, and these symptoms persist and become more severe, it is very important that you take charge of your health care personally. No matter what you are told, insist on a pelvic ultrasound, CA 125 blood test, and a pelvic examination by a gynecologist. This approach will not diagnose all ovarian cancers but it will in the vast majority of cases. If you do not seize the moment a year may go by before the diagnosis is made and a lot can happen to an ovarian cancer in a year. Reread the chapter "In Their Own Words" for a quick refresher course.

I was just diagnosed with a Stage III cancer of the ovary. How long has it been there?

I am almost always asked this question. It is usually followed by the semi-accusatory question, "Why wasn't it picked up earlier?" If you had a surgical procedure six months before your diagnosis and the ovaries were visualized and normal you might be able to say that the cancer occurred after that. A previous CT scan showing an ovarian tumor would be another way of timing this event. However, in the vast majority of cases, no one is ever able to know how long a cancer of the ovary has been present. Questions regarding whether or not the tumor is *fast growing* are equally unanswerable.

I have found that some patients fixate on events in their past medical care and assign blame because they feel that the cancer should have been discovered earlier. I try to help these patients to put this issue on a sidetrack because I do not think that ongoing anger related to this problem helps with the healing process. Modern medicine, particularly as it relates to the diagnosis of ovarian cancer, is far from an exact science.

If my mother and my sister had ovarian cancer what should I do?

The first thing you should do is seek the help of a trained genetic counselor. Genetic counseling is a unique health care service that provides information and support for people who are at risk for genetically linked cancers. It involves the evaluation of your family history, a risk assessment, and a discussion of available testing options. Your gynecologist should be alerted and you should have an annual pelvic ultrasound and CA-125 blood test. You should know that only 10 percent of ovarian cancer is genetically linked. But if you have a deleterious mutation on the BRCA 1 gene and you are of Ashkenazi descent, your chance of getting ovarian cancer is **70 percent!**

Since there is no way to test for ovarian cancer and you have a strong family history for this disease you might consider having your ovaries removed. This operation can now be done with minimally invasive surgery. The National Institutes of Health have recommended that women with two or more first degree relatives with ovarian cancer should have their ovaries removed when they have completed childbearing or at age 35. I have mentioned on a number of occasions how useless the CA 125 test is as a screening mechanism. However, with patients who are at high risk, I do order this test and if it is very elevated I feel obligated to perform at least a laparoscopy.

The whole issue of genetic testing is confusing. How about a few simple sentences to help me understand this problem?

The incidence of ovarian cancer is 1.4 percent in the general population but it increases to 40 percent with a deleterious mutation in the BRCA 1 gene and 10 to 15 percent with a mutation in the BRCA 2 gene.

If you are BRCA positive, there is a 50 percent chance that your children and siblings will test positive. You will have an increased risk of developing one or both of these cancers and you should be screened more often for both breast and ovarian cancer.

If you are BRCA negative, there will be no hereditary factors that would pertain to the development of ovarian cancer but you must remember that only 10 percent of all ovarian cancers are genetically based. If you test negative, it is possible that your children will test positive.

A significant number of Jewish women remain uninformed regarding their increased susceptibility to ovarian cancer, especially if they have had breast cancer. BRCA screening is more important for them than it is for the general population.

Why not just get my ovaries removed and end the problem?

One of my greatest teachers taught me that the ovary is the exact equivalent of the testicle and should be treated with equal respect! She also taught me that a male surgeon never encounters an ovary healthy enough to retain or a testicle diseased enough to remove! The removal of both testicles will reduce the incidence of testicular cancer to zero and yet I cannot imagine a line forming for such preventive medicine. The decision to have one's ovaries removed is as important as it is deeply personal and should be made only after considerable thought and discussion. Equality among gonads, while interesting in concept, is not relevant in the world of oncology as a cancer of the testicle is so easy to diagnose with treatment outcomes so vastly superior to what is seen in ovarian cancer.

I always tell my patients that I am very good at removing ovaries and very bad at putting them back. This is a preposterous statement calculated to imbue them with the irrevocability of their decision. A 70-year-old woman of Ashkenazi descent who has a deleterious mutation on the BRCA 1 gene and whose mother and sister have had ovarian cancer should have her ovaries removed without delay. However, most patients do not present with such overwhelming mandates and therefore much wisdom and compassion are required on the part of the attending physician. We should remember that these decisions are not emergencies and that a properly informed patient will almost always make the right decision if given enough time.

I am 26 years old with pelvic pain and a slightly elevated CA125—what should I do?

The vast majority of such patients will **not** have ovarian cancer. The CA 125 is mainly a test for inflammation and is frequently elevated in women with endometriosis and fibroid tumors of the uterus. A pelvic ultrasound should be done. In the absence of a suspicious mass you should be given the birth control pill and have an ultrasound and CA 125 repeated. This problem can always be resolved by performing a laparoscopy, which is the insertion of a camera through the navel. This allows not only visualization but also the opportunity to remove any pathology which may be causing the pain. This is where the experience of the physician plays such a major role. No one wants to have or perform surgery that is unnecessary. One should never take a trip to the operating room lightly. Although quite rare today, horrendous complications have occurred at the time of laparoscopic procedures.

The consumer of health care should be guided by one of surgery's great aphorisms; *a minor operation is an operation that is done on somebody else!* Please remember that the last person to agree to have an operation is a surgeon! They all ask, "What are the alternatives?"

There is at least a gallon of fluid in my abdomen—does this mean that I definitely have ovarian cancer?

Not necessarily! Meigs syndrome refers to a benign, solid tumor of the ovary accompanied by fluid in the abdomen and chest. A week prior to writing this chapter I operated on a 37-year-old woman with five liters of fluid in the abdomen and a CT scan showing a pelvic mass as well as a mass abutting the transverse colon. All of this proved to be benign endometriosis! People like this probably do very well in Las Vegas also.

Meigs syndrome is very rare and so a large fluid collection in the abdomen of a woman is a cancer of the ovary until proven otherwise and the appropriate workup should be initiated. A Stage IV cancer of the ovary may produce fluid in the abdomen and yet the ovaries can be normal in size and the ultrasound and CT scan may show only fluid! Whenever there is any doubt, a laparoscopy should be performed.

As mentioned earlier, the fluid can be removed on an outpatient basis by simply inserting a small catheter under ultrasound or CT guidance. The fluid should be sent to the cytology laboratory for analysis. There are two hugely important things to remember about this process: The fluid may contain **no** cancer cells whatsoever even though an advanced cancer of the ovary is present; cancer cells may be present, suggesting that the primary cancer is **not** an ovarian cancer. I encountered such a patient last month when the cytology report on the fluid submitted showed Krukenberg cells indicating a gastrointestinal primary.

She turned out to have a primary cancer of the appendix, even though the colonoscopy was negative. The large ovarian mass was a metastatic cancer *to* the ovary and not a cancer originating *in* the ovary. At the time of surgery, I took care of the ovarian mass and a colorectal surgeon did a right colon resection. She is now being treated by a medical oncologist with chemotherapy drugs which would never be used for ovarian cancer. There is no room for error in this work. Had she been treated for a cancer of the ovary, disaster would have devolved on the situation.

I have a large mass in my ovary. Who should operate on me?

Most ovarian masses are benign and can be handled very well by your gynecologist. If the CA 125 is normal and the CT scan does not show any evidence of metastatic disease there is usually no need for a gynecologic oncologist to become involved. However, (and this is where the confusion lies) a significant cancer of the ovary may be present even in such an apparently benign scenario, and so it becomes a call for both the patient and the gynecologist.

I personally feel that all such patients should have their surgery in an operating room where a gynecologic oncologist is only moments away. When this is not possible then the procedure should begin with a laparoscopy and the abdomen opened only if a cancer is not found. If a cancer is found then the operation should be terminated and the patient referred to a gynecologic oncologist. Let me introduce another aphorism: The best shot in cancer treatment is the first shot!

All gynecologic oncologists dread the summons to an operating room when a cancer of the ovary is a surprise finding. There is frequently a tiny bikini incision, the bowel has not been emptied prior to surgery and no studies were done to rule out the presence of metastatic disease. This is by no means a criticism of the original surgeon; rather, it is an indication of how difficult it is to diagnose ovarian cancer prior to surgery.

How does surgery for a cancer of the ovary differ from surgery for benign conditions?

In many ways! The uterus and both tubes and ovaries should be removed, a procedure particularly tragic for a young woman. The omentum and appendix should be removed and an attempt should be made to remove all of the cancer. This frequently involves the removal of the recto-sigmoid colon as well as part of the small intestine. Tumor implants on the liver and diaphragm are frequently present and need to be removed. Sometimes it is even necessary to remove a major portion of the diaphragm. Since ovarian cancer has access to the entire abdominal cavity, the masses can be anywhere and will need to be removed or destroyed with one of the new surgical vaporizing instruments.

Such a procedure should always be done by a gynecologic oncologist. General gynecologists are neither trained nor experienced in the performance of such surgery.

Will I need chemotherapy following surgery?

With very rare exception the use of chemotherapy will be absolutely necessary. Chemotherapy goes hand in hand with surgery and one without the other invariably dooms the patient to a recurrence. I am frequently asked if it is possible to wait and give chemotherapy if the tumor comes back. While this question is understandable, the golden opportunity to give the chemotherapy in a setting of *zero tumor burden*, which would exist immediately after surgery, would be lost. It is far less likely for chemotherapy to be effective in the presence of massive recurrent disease.

I find it helpful to discuss the probable need for chemotherapy at the same time that I discuss the surgical procedure. This tends to lessen the shock and depression that accompanies the immediate postoperative period as the bad news is delivered in one message and not incrementally.

I am being treated for ovarian cancer and I am BRCA positive. What should I do to prevent breast cancer?

If breast cancer were as difficult to diagnose as ovarian cancer the answer would be so simple—surgery as soon as possible! Women have two diametrically opposed choices and the decision is never an emergency. A mammogram and ultrasound can be done every six months. It would be extremely unusual for an advanced cancer of the breast to emerge in such a careful follow-up setting. The alternative would be a bilateral mastectomy with or without breast reconstruction.

In addition to the physical side of the surgical decision, there can be grave psychological problems. These women have just had extensive gynecologic surgery and are castrate and menopausal. The removal of both breasts is a bridge too far for many of them. However, some patients are vehemently proactive and sign up for the surgery almost immediately and others will not even discuss the surgical option. I advise my patients to see a genetic counselor and I refer them to a breast cancer center for follow-up. I emphasize that they have a choice and with respect to surgery the choice is irrevocable.

Nowhere in my career have I found time to be a more important issue. Such patients should read materials that dwell on both options and should seek other opinions when additional counsel will be of benefit. They should talk to patients who have and have not visited the surgical option while remembering that their personal histories may differ from those of other patients. It has been my experience that these women, armed with the correct information and counseled by experienced and caring members of the health care team, will inevitably make the proper decision if given enough time.

I am now in remission. If cancer of the ovary comes back where is it likely to appear? What will it do to me and how will it be treated?

These are universal questions even if they never enter the patient's consciousness. As we have seen, ovarian cancer can recur more than ten years after treatment has been stopped. The most likely location is within the abdominal cavity. Although sometimes there are no symptoms at all, what we see most often are cramping abdominal pain and bloating, the mirror image of the initial presentation. The recurrent tumor can vary from a large mass frequently attached to the recto-sigmoid colon to hundreds of small nodules scattered throughout the abdominal cavity.

If you get a recurrence, it will be of enormous help to you psychologically to know that you are not alone and that there are many such patients out there who would be very pleased to talk with you and guide you through these bleak and troubled waters. I have so often seen such encounters bring about a sense of calm and focus that I was only partially able to accomplish.

A PET/CT scan of the chest, abdomen, and pelvis should be done to document the extent of the recurrence, which can then be used to evaluate the success of subsequent treatment. Chemotherapy is mandatory and your physician will guide you as to whether a surgical procedure needs to be done prior to the resumption of chemotherapy. It is possible to make the boo-boo go away! You would think that after all these years in practice I could come up with better terminology to describe a recurrent ovarian cancer!

When should I get another opinion?

A second opinion is always appropriate when the patient or the family feels that it is a good idea. Under such circumstances the treating physician should see to it that the transfer is as seamless as possible and that the records are sent in a timely fashion. Most patients who seek another opinion will return to the care of the original physician. When opinions differ it will take a great deal of time to explain the disparate possibilities and to help the patient settle into the regimen that is eventually adopted.

A second opinion can occur with a simple phone call from one physician to another. However, there are times when the patient feels better if she can actually meet the physician who is providing the second opinion. Some advanced treatments are available only in a few centers, and, when appropriate, patients need to be informed of this.

I have had extensive surgery for cancer of the ovary and am in the middle of chemotherapy. When will I get my life back?

The return to a normal life is the common thread peculiar to patients' aspirations whether they are retired and work in their gardens or whether they are major executives in a big company. Most of my patients continue to work during chemotherapy and this provides at least the perception that things will soon get back to normal. I think it is important that they look forward to a specific date when the chemotherapy will be stopped and that some sort of celebration is planned around this event. One of the most important ways to expedite the beginning of a patient's return to normal is to have her meet several people who have undergone a similar journey many years ago, and whose appearance is a startling example of what is possible. You should never run out of either plans or dreams.

It is important that you be told that you are in great part responsible for the taking back of your life. However, it is hugely difficult in the beginning. Pain and weakness slow you down but the return to the *usual routine* is frequently an accomplishable goal. It's the cancer Olympics. Train! Train! I'll act as coach. I'll act as spiritual advisor. But you have to meet me halfway!

I have recurrent cancer of the ovary and the third regimen of chemotherapy has failed. Am I doomed?

Such situations are the most desperate that oncologists ever face. However, it is my opinion that the correct answer is to be found in the famous Broadway phrase, "It ain't necessarily so." A realist should balance that answer with the knowledge that most patients who fail three chemotherapy regimens will eventually die of their disease. The chance that the oncologist will be able to get rid of all the recurrent cancer with the use of treatment modalities available today is virtually zero. And yet we have all seen situations where the amount of tumor is significantly reduced and the patient is transposed to a homeostatic state. The tumor does not bother her and the oncologist is unable to produce further dents.

I am now able to extend this discussion along lines that I would have found inappropriate ten years ago. There has evolved in the past several years a body of work that will soon radically change the manner in which all cancers will be treated. You should read over the sections in this book that deal with the basic science behind these impending changes. If you live into the dawn of this long sought-after world, your personal survival statistics may change dramatically.

What I am going to discuss now is a work in progress. It is the result of more than thirty years of interacting with women who have been reduced to a state of helplessness and whose anger and despair are initially directionless. In several parts of this book I have mentioned the value of a therapist and under no circumstances do I assume even amateur status in this area. How to focus anger and what benefit might be derived from this process is a controversial subject and what follows is merely a fleeting thought.

Get Angry! Rage against the dying of the light! Transpose a familiar object into a symbol with which you can communicate. In the film *Castaway*, Tom Hanks lives for many years on a deserted island after his plane crashes. He turns a volleyball into a companion and names him *Wilson*. Wilson acts as confidante and therapist. Silly! Crazy! Who cares! Whatever works! However, when you are in remission, perhaps it would be wise to find a way to diminish rage and put Wilson back on the shelf.

Further study on this topic has informed me that this idea might not be as strange as it initially appeared to me. Child psychiatrists have utilized *play therapy* for many years. They encourage children to vent their rage by hitting objects that sometimes bear the image of a clown.

I have lost my uterus, tubes, and ovaries and have just finished chemotherapy for cancer of the ovary. Is my sex life finished?

Absolutely not! If it is unwise for you to take hormone replacement therapy, there are numerous non-hormonal ways of dealing with the menopause. Here is a list of things that gynecologists frequently recommend:

- Exercise
- Vitamin E
- Isoflavones
- Effexor
- Clonidene

The sensitivity of the clitoris is unchanged and sexuality frequently returns to its pre-treatment level, but this sometimes requires counseling for the patient as well as the partner.

One of the most important factors in the return of one's sexuality is the mindset that the cancer is in the past tense. Estrogen replacement therapy in patients who are being treated for ovarian cancer is somewhat controversial but many gynecologic oncologists will consider this, especially in young patients.

In a large survey, 70 percent of patients treated for a gynecologic cancer reported problems with sexual dysfunction. Concepts of body image, despair, and grief are contributing factors. We should remember that commonly prescribed medications such as anti-depressants, narcotics, and anti-emetics (drugs that combat nausea) might exert a negative impact on sexuality.

There are excellent centers that specialize in all aspects of sexual dysfunction following treatment for a gynecologic malignancy. They will take a complete history and they are very skilled in all aspects of this problem. I have found that it is necessary for me to ask about these issues as my patients will rarely volunteer this information. We are all in this together. There is no need for cancer to interrupt life's centrifugal dance!

Is it possible to get ovarian cancer after I have had both ovaries removed?

Unfortunately, the answer to this question is yes. There are times when a small remnant of an ovary is left behind and this can become malignant. However, in most cases the patient has developed a primary peritoneal cancer. The peritoneum is the lining of the abdomen, the last thing that a surgeon cuts through to enter the abdominal cavity. The ovary and the peritoneum arise from the same tissue during the first few weeks of pregnancy and so a cancer coming from the peritoneum is similar to a cancer coming from the ovary.

The patterns of spread are identical and what one sees in the operating room is the same. The microscopic examination of the tissue is indistinguishable from ovarian cancer and the treatment is the same. Strictly speaking, however, it is not really ovarian cancer. Needless to say, these patients are most unlucky. The removal of the ovaries almost always prevents such a cancer.

I have been in remission for more than four years. Every time that I get a pain, every time I cough or get a headache I think that the ovarian cancer has come back. How do I handle this?

You are certainly not alone in this repetitive intrusion into sanity and peace of mind. We have all heard the onerous imperative, *Physician, heal thyself!* May I be permitted a descent into audacity and suggest something as novel as it is, perhaps, annoying? *Patient, heal thyself!* This may not be as flippant and insouciant a remark as it appears to be. Some patients have a more finely tuned immune engine that allows a cancer to be more easily placed into the past tense and others have a more finely honed emotional and personal matrix that allows for an easier approach to this terrifying disease. Our psyches are as disparate as our facial features and there is no universal *modus operandi* that helps everyone to cope with these very real and horrific issues.

I have mentioned compartmentalizing fear into four fifteen-minute periods each day. I have also suggested the use of a calendar to inscribe future events that will transpose you to places of joy with people you love. Why not try something different? Something that is unique to you! There is an 800-pound gorilla in your life and he has just asked you for the last dance. Use the extraordinary power of your mind and imagination to turn the gorilla first into a howling monkey and then into a mouse. Turn the intruder into something that is beneath you and then rise up and laugh at it. That is the ultimate degradation and it is *you* who are now the degrader! I just thought of this, and if I could think of this, then you can think of something better, something that will work for you! It has been my experience that therapists are not successful unless the patient does most of the work.

26

HEY BUD, CAN YOU SPARE 100K— IT'S FOR A GOOD CAUSE?

Be calm and strong and patient. Meet failure and disappointment with courage. Rise superior to the trials of life, and never give in to hopelessness or despair. In danger, in adversity, cling to your principles and ideals.

Aequanimitas!

—Sir William Osler

MY FATHER WAS a physician in New York City for many years and his office was located in an elegant old building called Medical Chambers. It was on 54th Street between Lexington and Third avenues and has long ago succumbed to a drab glass monstrosity. An old, blind gentleman stood at the entrance to his office building and sold pencils for a nickel apiece. My father never entered the building without giving him a nickel and he would never take a pencil. He was stopped in his tracks when, after many years, this apparent blind man said to my father, "I hate to complain, Doc, but the pencils are now a dime!"

This rather droll *non sequitur* was chosen to point out that medical research is much more expensive than it used to be. When Banting and Best conducted experiments on the pancreases of dogs, which eventually led to the production of insulin, the total bill encompassed the cost of dog food and some anesthetic drugs. Things have changed somewhat as it is unusual for us to order a piece of equipment that costs less than $100,000! Each part of the microarray puzzle generates huge amounts of data, which must be analyzed in mainframe computers. In addition to all of this, the Ovarian Cancer Institute must pay the salaries of our wonderful research staff. I very wisely stay out of the basic science aspect of our work and confine my efforts to the pristine collection and storage of tissue, serum, and data, and I leave the research in the capable hands of John McDonald. I have one other job for which neither medical school nor the Jesuits prepared me. I must raise the money to pay for all of this.

No one is lucky in everything! I have a wonderful family, work that gives me the illusion of accomplishment, and an extraordinary hospital in which to do that work. And, of course, I have as a partner in this venture a research scientist of the colossal stature of John McDonald. It is the art of relieving foundations of their money that continues to elude me. I am always so well received by these institutions. I am polite and both well mannered and well dressed. I state the mission and the dire needs of the Ovarian Cancer Institute with an impassioned grace tinged with a dash of pathos, and I always exit with the feeling that they could not possibly turn me down.

For some reason it is always exactly two weeks that go by before I receive *the* letter. All foundations seem to have taken the same course in the subtle art of graceful rejection. The first paragraph tells me how pleased they were to meet me and how important and exciting they find my work. The second paragraph explains, with an appropriate level of tragic regret, that our work does not fall within their "giving philosophy." However, it is the third paragraph that represents the twisting of the bejeweled dagger. "Dr. Benigno, we find your work so interesting and we hope that you will continue to keep us apprised of its progress!" Oh, to hear those beautiful and inspiring words, "Benigno, the entire board of this foundation considers you a worthless ass. Here's a cool million, now go away and don't ever come back!"

Desperation is a word that is familiar to all who run a cancer research institute and who are responsible for its funding. The balance in the checkbook is dwindling and no new sources of revenue are on the horizon. I was in such a state several years ago when someone brought me the dossiers of several wealthy women who were famous for giving large amounts of money to charitable causes. Their pictures were included and one of them caught my attention. When I looked up her original name I realized that I not only knew her when I was a young man, I had actually attended her wedding. This was the opportunity that I was waiting for—the chance that I would at last get the *big* check.

It took me hours to compose the letter, and, much against my better judgment, it ended with this most absurd sentence: "The memory of your grace and beauty lingers with me to this very day!" This bombastic statement was a bit over the top even for me, and should serve as an example to young researchers of how *not* to raise money. I justified it at the time by saying to myself that if all is fair in love and war, so all is excusable in the funding of a large cancer institute. It was exactly two weeks later, and guess what? I received *the* letter. It was a mirror image of all of the others only this one had a somewhat annoying personal touch. Her secretary had penciled in a message beneath the signature. "*Nice try, Doc!*" I disagree with the terminology. It was not a nice try. It was a noble try. The old full-court press!

I think that it was in *The Old Man and the Sea* where Ernest Hemingway wrote these famous words, "Man was not made for defeat. Man can be destroyed but he can never be defeated." That is all well and good, but Hemingway never had to fund cancer research in this financial climate. I need to convert a nice try into a successful try. We have enough funding to complete the research on our diagnostic test. We need considerably more money to complete the research on our stem cell project.

Ovarian Cycle is a charitable organization dedicated to funding research for this disease and we recently learned that they have earmarked $72,000 for the Ovarian Cancer Institute. Atlanta's famous Bacchanalia Restaurant will open its gracious doors for a major fundraising event for us. Just last week I received a letter from a New York law firm informing me that one of their clients was going to send us a check for $50,000! Not only was she not a patient but I had never heard of her before. Evidently she became aware of our work and decided, out of the blue, to fund it. That is exactly the kind of letter I like to receive from a law firm. Who knows, maybe my luck is changing!

27

THE TEST—
THE WAITING
GAME CONTINUES

*Twenty years from now you will be more
disappointed by the things that you didn't do than
by the ones you did do. So throw off the bowlines.
Sail away from the safe harbor. Catch the trade
winds in your sails. Explore. Dream. Discover.*

—Mark Twain

THERE IS NO other way to describe it. The final analysis
of our data, the work of more than ten years, was in limbo.
Although we had established that metabolic profiling could
distinguish ovarian cancer sera from normal sera, we did not
know the specific molecular identity of the diagnostic metabolites. We only knew them as mass/charge ratios. Since
our original publication, the machine in the laboratory and
the personnel responsible for calibrating the machine had
changed, and it became absolutely necessary that we learn the
identity of these diagnostic features. This was of great impor-

tance since the thirty Stage I samples we had purchased had enough serum for only one testing process.

Once the calibration of the new mass spectrometer is completed and the new personnel are familiar with its intricacies, we will begin the laborious work necessary to verify old results and run all of the serum specimens from the Stage I cancers. After this, we will have to see if the *peaks* produced by the mass spectrometer can be qualified in such a way that a company would be interested in becoming involved in this process. It would be impossible for us to do this on our own. Even if our data proves to be as wonderful as we think that it is, we will have to jump through the hoops of publication and FDA approval. It is not going to be as smooth and easy as I had anticipated.

I began writing this book a year ago and fully expected to be able to announce the arrival of a diagnostic test in the last chapter. While I think that this test will soon be a reality, it has not arrived yet. It is the most tantalizing piece of work that I have ever been involved in. There is no more appropriate adjective. Aldous Huxley once wrote:

> *"There are things known and there are things unknown,*
> *and in between are the doors of perception."*

Well, I just *know* that this test is everything that I have come to believe it is. 100 percent sensitive and 100 percent specific, done on a single drop of blood and costing fifty cents! I have the key; I just need to find the door!

In the meantime, I have to sit back and wait for all of this to unravel. No more specimens are needed and all of the data has been entered into the computer. It is time for the surgeon to stay out of all of this and simply wait. It reminds me of the opening of the famous film *Casablanca*. The Second World War is raging and everybody wants to get out of Casablanca and there are so few exit visas. As the plane is taking off for Lisbon, carrying just a few lucky passengers, the melodramatic voiceover says, "And they waited, and waited, and waited." Once again I feel stranded in a great waste of tedious disoccupation.

I have decided to send the manuscript off to the publisher. Hopefully a second edition will soon follow with a chapter that I am unfortunately not able to write at the present time.

28

DANA—THE FINALE

Only one ship is seeking us, a black-
Sailed unfamiliar, towing at her back
A huge and birdless silence. In her wake
No waters breed or break.

—Philip Larkin

How should I not be glad to contemplate
the clouds clearing beyond the dormer window
and a high tide reflected on the ceiling?
There will be dying, there will be dying,
but there is no need to go into that.
The poems flow from the hand unbidden
and the hidden source is the watchful heart.
The sun rises in spite of everything
and the far cities are beautiful and bright.
I lie here in a riot of sunlight
Watching the day break and the clouds flying.
Everything is going to be all right.

—Derek Mahon
"Everything Is Going to Be All Right"

I THINK IT fitting that this book should end the way in which it began—with the protagonist at center stage. Oncology success stories tend to fade and reside in a subliminal Neverland; visual images of our failures are somehow always with us. Dana did well for quite some time following the last and most extensive of her surgical procedures, but then, like a coda in a sonata, the theme presented itself again, with the return of symptoms and CT evidence of recurrent disease.

The silence on both our parts spoke volumes and she finally asked me if she was going to die. I told her that it was very likely. I did not tell her what I knew only too well, that the correct answer was a resounding yes! The twenty-five years of our relationship interdicted, at that time, my ability to confer absolute finality to the question asked. I realize that the incompletely answered question can be the greatest of lies, but I ask the reader to understand the difficulty of the situation. Sometimes even oncologists need a breather.

Since Dana's tumor was estrogen receptor positive I gave her a prescription for Arimidex, which is a drug that attacks tumor tissue rich in estrogen. It is widely used in some breast cancers and has been used in the treatment of ovarian cancer for many years. It had little chance of making a meaningful and lasting difference, but there was a possibility that it could temporarily arrest the growth of the tumor. It consisted of a single pill once a day with few if any side effects. We both felt that it would be worth a try.

She who had responded previously to every imaginable form of therapy quickly faded before my eyes as if the dimmer switch of a bright light had been quickly slid down to the off position. It had been twenty-five years, a quarter of a century, and she simply gave up, signed up with Hospice, went home, and died. It is not uncommon for some patients to become part of the physician's extended family and in her case I lost not only a patient but also a friend.

I have a rule that I had never broken before. No funerals, because funerals are a bridge too far! I broke this rule in her case for two reasons; twenty-five years is a long time, and, more importantly, she had asked me to attend her funeral. The cathedral was packed, the tributes glowing, and mixed with the sadness and loneliness was a naked question. **Why?**

Is it too outlandish to hope that the test that we are in the process of developing might one day prevent not only such a death, but also the twenty-five years of anxiety and all of the horrific treatments that she had to endure? No one who gets an annual Pap smear should ever die of cervical cancer. Will be able to say the same about ovarian cancer when this test is finally available?

EPILOGUE

FEW THINGS RIVAL death in the poet's armamentarium of metaphors. Although we are assured of our own impending demise intellectually, we don't seem to be able to process such a concept as it pertains to ourselves. It is the arrival of the third recurrence that blasts suspension of reality into real time. If life is a banquet then cancer takes away the knife and fork and pulls the chair out from under us. This seems to be just as annoying for the octogenarian having dessert as it is for the adolescent about to eat the appetizer.

I disagree vehemently with the concept that one's approach to death can be divided into several neatly defined stages that progress in numerical order. In my experience, these stages are as random and repetitive as the cell divisions that characterize the cancer itself. Denial and anger never seem to really go away; they are simply not expressed as often. Who could possibly have several operations and multiple regimens of chemotherapy and stop being angry or at times not feel that this is a bad play and I am not really in it?

I have found the CA 125 blood test to be a stagnating influence in a patient's life. After treatment has been stopped and the patient is in a follow-up mode, this test is usually ordered every three months. Patients seem to live for the next report, becoming understandably agitated as the blood is drawn and relax once again only when the result has come back and is normal. I try to understand the angst that accompanies a rise in a CA 125 test from a four to a five and have learned that no fear in such patients should be taken lightly. I can think of no laboratory test that produces more distress and anxiety. I often wonder if patients would do better if I simply stopped ordering it!

Depression is a far more difficult issue than I imagined when I was a young oncologist. I have to continually remind myself that when the patient comes into the office she has spent a considerable amount of time preparing for the visit both physically and emotionally, and that the reality of her return home might be a much different scenario. Therapists and antidepressant medications have their place, but I have come to believe that it is the patient's personal treating oncologist who can put up a roadblock barring an encounter with the edge of nothingness. As far as acceptance is concerned, I frequently see that just before the comatose state, and sometimes not even then.

Depression in a cancer patient can take many forms and one of the most interesting is survivor's guilt. If I don't know why some patients do well and others do not, how is it possible for patients to know? The open chemotherapy suite is a marvelous instrument of healing as it confers on the patient the idea that she is not alone. Patients bond with one another and the death of one of them produces fear and anxiety in the survivors. Such a death produces another interesting phenomenon, which I call *the other shoe syndrome*. Patients who "graduate" from chemotherapy at the same time frequently come to know each other very well and invariably keep in touch. When they are informed of the death of one of their cohorts/friends, they go through a grieving process which includes waiting for the news of *their* recurrence. This is one of the bizarre fruits in the cornucopia of grief.

The oncologist who has a standard speech for all patients who are afraid and depressed will be of help only 5 percent of the time. As treatment gravitates to the personalized approach so should the conversations that accompany the treatment. We all realize that some patients require more time than others, especially in the beginning of the relationship. The one universal fear among all of these patients is usually expressed early on and it is contained in the question, "Am I going to die?"

There are many ways to respond to this question. I frequently tell them that we are all going to die and my sacred responsibility is to see to it that they do not die of ovarian cancer. I also tell them that if it recurs and is not cured, it can sometimes be converted to a chronic disease state. I mention the extraordinary research being done at the present time—

research that will eventually make all of the surgery and chemotherapy now required to get rid of cancer seem barbaric by comparison. I tell them that the cavalry has left the fort! I conclude by telling them that their names are on the invite list to my retirement party in twenty years: Ritz-Carlton Hotel, black tie! No gifts, please!

In reading over this manuscript it occurred to me that the recounting of the patients' histories tended to dwell on those patients who did poorly. There are several reasons for this: First of all, these are the people that the oncologist sees much more frequently than those who are in remission; their stories are more dramatic and replete with an unbearable pathos; and, lastly, they imbue us with the sheer frailty of the human condition and invite us to examine our own mortality. There are so many patients who have done well and after five years they are seen only every six months and no longer live for their next CA 125! Without exception they serve in the trenches when called upon to counsel newly diagnosed patients and provide a pulse of enthusiasm and hope that a whole platoon of oncologists could not match. Let me end on a happy note by telling you of a patient who did so very well despite the fact that the deck was stacked against her

PATRICIA

This extremely bright and very well-dressed woman came into my office complaining of the sudden onset of vague, cramping abdominal pain and the sense of being "full" after a few bites of food. I felt not only a mass filling the pelvis, but also a mass in the upper abdomen. The CA125 was elevated and the CT scan was compatible with an advanced cancer of the ovary. I will never forget the equanimity with which she responded to the pieces of information that eventually led to the bald declarative sentence, "You almost certainly have an advanced cancer of the ovary and you will need an extensive surgical procedure." She told me that she had a feeling that I was going to tell her that and declined a second opinion and wanted the surgery scheduled as soon as possible.

The operation removed the tumors but required the removal of the sigmoid colon and the upper rectum along with a rejoining of the colon with a stapling device. All visible tumor was removed, which is one of the most important prognostic factors. She tolerated six courses of chemotherapy better than most patients half her age and subsequent examinations, CT scans, and CA 125s have been normal. She came into the office last month encouraging me to read a book titled *The Hare with Amber Eyes.* Among her many pet projects is the desire to improve my education. I should mention that her surgery was seven years ago!

As I grow older I have noticed a strange tendency to continue to shoulder the blame when things go wrong but to assume only partial credit when things go well. As a young surgeon I would have taken full credit for Patricia's wonderful recovery, but extensive experience and my involvement in the basic science research at the Ovarian Cancer Institute have taught me that the internal combustion of my patient's immune engine is at least as important as the surgery and chemotherapy that I provide. In the near future we will be able to fine-tune this immune engine and allow it to participate more fully in the therapeutic process. Scientists and oncologists will be able to tap into the personal structure of an individual cancer process and select a personalized treatment plan based on the very molecular configuration of the malignancy. I call this *designer treatment*. Giorgio Armani does cancer therapy!

What is wrong with the author asking the reader a question? Why don't all patients with ovarian cancer do as well as Patricia? Well, maybe they all will some day and perhaps that day is sooner at hand than most of us realize. The epilogue of a book that describes cancer in all of its dreariness and includes graphic descriptions of those who have died of this disease should end on the expectation that the treatments described are on the way out. Please remember that the adjective *barbaric* has been used to describe current, state-of-the-art modalities of treatment.

Washington University has one of the world's leading genetic research departments. One of their young and very talented scientists developed acute lymphoblastic leukemia and was deteriorating fast. No known treatment could help him and, furthermore, the complete genetic composition of this cancer had never been investigated.

As reported in a *New York Times* article recently, Dr. Timothy Levy, the associate director of the university's genomic institute, called his research team together and told them to think *outside the box*. They did something that had never been done with this disease before. They fully sequenced the genes of his cancer cells and compared the results to the sequencing of his normal cells. After running one of the sequencing machines around the clock, they finally found the problem. One of the genes was in overdrive and was producing huge amounts of a protein that appeared to be causing the cancer's growth. They became aware of a new drug that might shut down this malfunctioning gene. This drug, unfortunately, had been tested and approved only for advanced kidney cancer!

This young researcher became the first person ever to take this drug for acute lymphoblastic leukemia, and to everyone's amazement, he went into immediate remission and has remained free of disease ever since. The name of the drug is *sunitinib* and we must remember that this was the first time that it was ever used for anything except advanced kidney disease.

It doesn't take an expert to realize that this was an *inside job*. If this had been Jane Blow from Lubbock, Texas, the usual drugs would have been given with the usual outcome. Earlier in the book it was mentioned that some people believe that the cure for cancer has been discovered already but not yet recognized. While I do not believe that to be true, this gene sequencing story may prove to be a giant step forward. What happened to this young scientist contains a very powerful message for all of us.

One woman's ovarian cancer may have an entirely different genetic composition than another woman's ovarian cancer. Indeed, that woman's ovarian cancer might have more in common, with respect to genetic composition, with some man's pancreatic cancer. I am stressing these facts to point out that there are many drugs currently available in the treatment of cancer, and drugs are chosen along certain strict guidelines. Sunitinib would never have been chosen for this patient's leukemia unless the genetic sequencing had elucidated the overproduction of a protein that this drug was exquisitely positioned to turn off. Is it time to subject the genetic composition of every cancer to such intense sequencing prior to recommending a course of chemotherapy? It would be very expensive, but then again, so are wars!

Let me end by paraphrasing something that the great Susan Sontag once said. Death is inevitable but degradation is not on the dance card.

ABOUT THE AUTHOR

BENEDICT B. BENIGNO, M.D., is a board certified gynecologic oncologist and the founder and chief executive officer of the Ovarian Cancer Institute. He currently serves as principal investigator for numerous clinical trials for ovarian cancer and has authored many scientific articles in peer review journals. He is the director of gynecologic oncology as well as the director of research at Northside Hospital in Atlanta, Georgia.

He is a graduate of the Georgetown University School of Medicine and completed a residency in obstetrics and gynecology at Saint Vincent's Hospital and Medical center in New York City. He did fellowship training in gynecologic oncology at the Emory University School of Medicine and MD Anderson Cancer Center at the University of Texas in Houston.

As a young surgeon he was appointed visiting professor at the University Medical School in Saigon, South Vietnam, where he spent three years during the war setting up a residency training program in obstetrics and gynecology. He then became a professor in the department of gynecology and obstetrics at the Emory University School of Medicine, where he served as director of gynecologic oncology. He subsequently founded University Gynecologic Oncology and serves as its president. It is a practice composed of four board-certified gynecologic oncologists based at Northside Hospital.

He is married and has three children.

CPSIA information can be obtained at www.ICGtesting.com
Printed in the USA
LVOW06s2033181013

357601LV00031B/2063/P